LIVING THE
REIKI

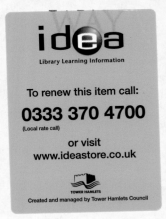

WITHDRAWN

LIVING THE
REIKI
WAY

*Traditional Principles
for Living Today*

PENELOPE QUEST

piatkus

PIATKUS

First published in Great Britain in 2008 by Piatkus Books
This paperback edition published in 2010 by Piatkus

3 5 7 9 10 8 6 4 2

A CIP catalogue record for this book
is available from the British Library.

ISBN 978-0-7499-2933-6

Typeset in Bembo by Action Publishing Technology Ltd, Gloucester
Printed and bound by CPI Group (UK) Ltd, Croydon, CR0 4YY

Papers used by Piatkus are from well-managed forests
and other responsible sources.

MIX
Paper from
responsible sources
FSC® C104740

Piatkus
An imprint of
Little, Brown Book Group
Carmelite House
50 Victoria Embankment
London EC4Y 0DZ

An Hachette UK Company
www.hachette.co.uk

www.piatkus.co.uk

This book is dedicated to my mother,
Irene Monica Harris (1913–1999), who taught
me to appreciate life and live it my way.

CONTENTS

ACKNOWLEDGEMENTS

I would like to express my heartfelt gratitude to the many people who have helped, directly or indirectly, with this book, especially to my friend Revd Simon John Barlow, for allowing me to adapt some of the material we wrote together for our workshops on consciousness, meditation and visualization. I would also like to thank my son Chris and daughter Kathy for their unfailing love and support in everything I do, and my many Reiki friends and students for the love and learning they have brought me. In addition, thank you to Helen, Gill, Krystyna and Rebecca from Piatkus, for their enthusiasm and help, and to my readers for all the wonderful emails you send me, which are always greatly appreciated and very inspiring.

Of course, special thanks go to my Reiki teachers Kristin Bonney, William Lee Rand, Andy Bowling, Richard Rivard and Robert Jefford, who have been so instrumental in my own Reiki journey. Thanks also go to the many other teachers and writers who have advanced my knowledge and experience in the various other subjects, such as psychology, NLP, EFT, abundance theory, meditation and spiritual development, which have been such a useful foundation for writing this book.

INTRODUCTION

Reiki has been an essential part of my life since 1991 when I attended my first Reiki course, and I have been trying to 'live the Reiki way' ever since. I worked part-time as a Reiki practitioner for a number of years, alongside my work as a lecturer and senior manager in a college, and in 1994 I qualified as a Reiki Master – the term that describes a teacher of Reiki. By 1996 I knew that practising and teaching Reiki was what I really wanted to do, so I left my job in order to devote more time to teaching and writing about Reiki.

However, along the way, in addition to learning more and gaining further qualifications in Reiki and writing a number of books on the subject, I have followed many other interests and gained knowledge and experience in a wide range of topics, including psychology, meditation and visualization, Neuro Linguistic Programming (NLP), Emotional Freedom Technique (EFT), Native American and Celtic shamanism, abundance theory and cosmic ordering, and other areas of study that promote under-standing, personal growth and a holistic view of the person. My special interest in healing has also led me to learn a number of other healing methods, such as Hawaiian Huna and Karuna Reiki®, and recently I added to my academic qualifications by gaining a Masters degree in Health and Healing Science.

It was this wide-ranging background that led me to want to write a book about living with the Reiki principles in today's hectic world. For me, living the Reiki way hasn't just been about Reiki, although Reiki has certainly been the most important aspect of my personal spiritual and healing journey for nearly twenty years. But I believe that Reiki has also been instrumental in guiding me to other methods for personal growth and spiritual development, as well as to various self-help techniques for my own healing, and this is why I have incorporated some of these within this book. While I think Reiki is fantastic, I am aware that it isn't the only way forward, so I wanted to present some other methods for people to explore. Sometimes Reiki is all you need, and at other times another method, such as NLP, EFT, or working through a visualization, will help to produce the shift in perception or energy you need to help you to deal with a problem.

Nearly a century ago Dr Mikao Usui, the founder of the healing system we call Reiki, encouraged his students to live by the following precepts:

Just for today, do not anger, do not worry, be filled with gratitude, devote yourself to your work, and be kind to people.

Reiki students today are advised to live by the same principles, but perhaps these present even more of a challenge in the 21st century. Nevertheless, I believe they can be a great help and support to people in their everyday lives, as well as offering a way to a more spiritual path of personal growth.

Living the Reiki Way isn't just intended for people who already use Reiki, although I hope they will find plenty within its pages that is both helpful and inspiring. It is a book for anyone interested in personal growth and spiritual development – so whether you've just done your first Reiki course, or have practised or taught Reiki for years, or even if this is the first you've heard about Reiki, you will find something here for you.

Living the Reiki Way includes suggestions for using Reiki (or healing energy) to help you to cope with strong emotions like anger, or to understand how being grateful can bring a lot of joy and happiness into your life – although these methods can only be employed by those who have undertaken at least one Reiki course. However, there are plenty of other techniques that anyone can use, whether they have learned Reiki or not. These include meditations, visualizations and self-help techniques utilizing NLP and EFT, all of which you will find beneficial.

For those who may not know very much about Reiki, Chapter 1 covers the Reiki basics, including what Reiki is, where it originated, how it works, what a Reiki treatment consists of, what effects Reiki can have and how you can learn to do Reiki yourself. If you need more detailed information about Reiki, you will find it in my other books – *The Basics of Reiki, Reiki for Life* and *Self-healing with Reiki* (see Further Reading, page 255).

While this is therefore a book based on Reiki, it embraces a great deal more than Reiki alone: it provides information, advice and useful techniques to help you navigate through strong emotions, negative thinking habits, fear, worry, lack of self-belief and other issues that might be holding you back from achieving your true potential. It offers principles for living today that are every bit as vital as they were when Dr Usui was alive, and that can help you to change, let go of destructive patterns of thinking and feeling, and develop your own positive attitudes, beliefs, concepts and philosophy for life.

Living the Reiki Way is about living thoughtfully, kindly, generously, gratefully, calmly, confidently, considerately, diligently, conscientiously and happily. If those are aspects you would like to demonstrate in your life, read on!

part one

REIKI BASICS

The secret method of inviting happiness;
The wonderful medicine for all diseases.

Mikao Usui

chapter one

WHAT IS REIKI?

This book is about living the Reiki way, or, in other words, living with the Reiki Principles in today's modern world. Anyone who has taken part in a Reiki course or workshop will know what the Reiki Principles are, but there may be readers of this book who haven't heard of them before, and perhaps, more to the point, don't really know what Reiki is. To set the scene, in this chapter I describe briefly what Reiki is and where it came from – this will make other chapters in this book easier to understand. However, if you have already read one of my other books, especially *The Basics of Reiki* or *Reiki for Life*, or have taken part in a Reiki course, you can probably skip this chapter and go straight to Chapter 2. For anyone else, please read on!

THE ORIGINS OF REIKI

We may never know the exact origins of Reiki as a healing system, but it probably dates back at least 2,500 years, as we know that the Buddha used something similar, and it is likely to be even older than that. However, the healing system we use today in the West, which we call Reiki, was developed initially in the 1920s by Dr Mikao Usui (1865–1926), a Buddhist priest in Japan, and further developed by one of his students, Dr Chujiro Hayashi (1879–1940), who passed his teachings on between 1936 and 1938 to a Hawaiian woman of Japanese parentage, Mrs Hawayo Takata (1900–1980). She was responsible for bringing the teachings to the West, initially to Hawaii, the USA and Canada, and through the 22 teachers (Reiki Masters) she taught between 1972 and 1980 to the rest of the Western world.

WHAT IS REIKI?

The way in which Reiki is seen in the West today is primarily as a form of complementary therapy – a safe, gentle, non-intrusive, hands-on healing technique that uses spiritual energy (the Japanese word *reiki* means spiritual energy or universal life-force energy) to treat physical ailments. It is, however, much more than a physical therapy; it is a holistic system for balancing, healing and harmonizing all aspects of the person – body, mind, emotions and spirit – promoting relaxation and a sense of well-being.

It is therefore healing in its most all-encompassing sense – healing the physical, emotional, psychological and spiritual aspects enables a person to become whole, or 'holy' in what was possibly the original sense of the word. Unlike other complementary or alternative therapies, the practice of Reiki is also a spiritual discipline that includes meditation, energy-cleansing techniques and spiritual principles for living, and practitioners are encouraged to use Reiki on themselves daily not only for self-healing, but also to increase self-awareness, personal growth and spiritual development.

THE WAY REIKI WORKS

Life-force energy (Ki or Chi) flows within the physical body through energy centres called chakras and pathways called meridians, as well as flowing around the body in a field of energy called the aura. This energy field responds to everything we think, say, feel and experience, and it becomes disrupted or blocked whenever we consciously or unconsciously accept and absorb negative words, thoughts, feelings or experiences. If these blockages are not dispersed, their energy can gradually become more dense, which is when they can transform into physical illnesses. Reiki is a spiritual energy vibrating at a very high rate that helps to break through these blockages, flowing through all the affected parts of the aura and the physical body, charging them with positive energy and raising the vibratory level of the whole energy field. It clears and balances the chakras, and straightens the energy pathways (meridians), allowing the life force to flow in a healthy and natural way around the whole body. This strengthens and accelerates the body's own natural ability to heal itself, and opens the mind, emotions and spirit to an acceptance and understanding of the causative issues that have led to 'dis-ease' in both the physical and energy bodies.

Because Reiki is guided by a Higher Intelligence (God, the Universe, your Soul or Higher Self, or whatever description you feel comfortable with), it always finds its way to the areas of the physical body and/or the energy body most in need of healing, without any conscious direction from either the healer or the person being healed, and it adjusts to suit the recipient, so that each person receives as much or as little healing as they need.

A REIKI TREATMENT

Many people first experience Reiki when they receive a Reiki treatment from a holistic practitioner. Reiki treatments take about an hour, and are usually carried out with you lying comfortably on a therapy couch, covered with a soft blanket. You remain fully clothed (except for shoes and coat), and the practitioner's hands are placed and held still for 3–5 minutes in each of about 12 specific positions over your head and body. There is no pressure, manipulation or massage, and no sensitive or intimate areas of the body need to be touched.

The most usual hand positions are:

◆ Four on the head – the back of the head, over the ears or temples, over the eyes and on either side of the neck.
◆ Four on the front of the body – the upper chest, solar plexus, navel area and pelvic area.
◆ Four on the back of the body – the shoulders, middle of the back, waist level and buttocks.

You usually feel very relaxed, warm and peaceful as the energy flows through you – people often fall asleep during the treatment – although sometimes you might feel heat, coolness or tingles where the practitioner's hands are placed (this is quite normal). It is also quite normal for people to feel a bit emotional sometimes, as the Reiki releases blocked energy and brings to the surface old issues and patterns to be released, so memories might come flooding back. After a treatment some people feel super-energized, while others feel very tranquil and sleepy.

TREATING YOURSELF WITH REIKI

Once you have learned how to use Reiki, being able to treat yourself is one of its great advantages, because it encourages you to take responsibility for yourself and your own health and well-being, and most Reiki practitioners use it on themselves every day. A full self-treatment involves the same 12 or more hand positions on your head and body as those described above, but you can also give yourself Reiki at other times – while watching television, for example – by simply placing your hands on any part of your body and holding them there for as long as it feels comfortable.

Reiki can also be successfully incorporated into many of the healing arts practised by health professionals, such as reflexology, aromatherapy, shiatsu, osteopathy, etc, because the Reiki energy can simply flow out of the practitioner's hands during the treatment, to promote even greater healing effects.

THE EFFECTS OF REIKI

Most people who go for a Reiki treatment want help with a specific physical problem, from frequent headaches or a frozen shoulder, to more serious complaints, although some simply want to be able to relax and cope better with the stresses of modern life – you don't have to be ill to benefit from Reiki! The potential with Reiki is unlimited, so anything can be treated, but it is important to rid yourself of specific expectations of what it will do, and how fast it will perform. Many physical symptoms can be eased very quickly, while others may need a lot of Reiki before starting to respond, but it is essential to remember that it is *your own body* that is actually doing the healing.

The human body has an amazing ability to regenerate itself, as most of the cells in your body are replaced each year, which is why physical healing can happen – as an example, if you cut yourself, new skin cells are produced to heal the cut. Some people report amazing, even miraculous, effects from Reiki treatments, but 'healing' is not *always* the same as 'curing', although we tend to use the words interchangeably, which creates misunderstanding. Healing doesn't always occur on the physical level first. Because Reiki works holistically, it may be that healing needs to happen first at the emotional level, with the releasing of anger, guilt or hatred, or it may be required first at the mental level, releasing negative thoughts, concepts or attitudes, or at the spiritual level, developing self-awareness, self-understanding and self-love, before the physical symptoms can be addressed.

If you are open-minded and willing to receive the

Reiki (belief in it is not a prerequisite) healing *will* take place, although it may not always be in quite the way you expect – Reiki goes where it is needed, not always where you want it to go! Ultimately, if you want the healing to be permanent you have to take responsibility for healing the cause. This may mean changing how you think or the way you relate to other people, or even altering your whole lifestyle, from your diet and home environment to your close relationships, job or career. Surprisingly, perhaps, Reiki can help with these adjustments too, allowing you to approach the changes in a relaxed way.

LEARNING HOW TO USE REIKI

Reiki is probably the simplest and easiest holistic healing method available to us, so anyone can learn to use it, whatever their age or gender, religion or origin. No specific previous knowledge or experience is required – only a desire to learn, willingness to let this healing energy flow through you and a little time to attend your first course. The ability to channel Reiki can only be acquired by being transferred to the student by a quali- fied Reiki Master (Teacher) in a special ceremony during a Reiki course, called an attunement, which is a form of spiritual empowerment based on ancient Buddhist tech- niques. This attunement process makes Reiki unique and is the reason why the ability to heal can be developed so quickly yet so permanently. It activates a Reiki channel through which the Reiki healing energy can flow, and once you have been attuned you will be able to use Reiki for the rest of your life – the ability to channel Reiki doesn't wear off or wear out. From then on, whenever you intend to use Reiki, simply thinking about it, or holding your hands out in readiness to use it on yourself or someone else, will activate the flow of Reiki energy.

There are three levels of training, usually referred to as 'degrees'. These do not refer to (or confer) any academic level or qualification; they are just used to describe the different training levels.

- At First Degree, which can be a one- or two-day course, you normally receive four 'attunements', which gradually open up your inner healing channel, allowing Reiki to flow through. The emphasis at this level is on self-healing, although you will also be taught how to carry out a treatment on family, friends and animals.

- The Second Degree course usually takes one or two days, and includes another attunement that enables you to access even more Reiki. You learn three sacred symbols (shapes that you draw in the air with your hand) and their mantras (sacred names). These are called the Distant (Connection) symbol that allows you to connect with anyone or anything in any time or space; the Harmony (Mental and Emotional) symbol that helps to bring peace and harmony to a person, animal or situation; and the Power (Focus) symbol that brings extra Reiki energy into whatever it is focused upon. You will also learn some special ways of using them, including a form of distant healing that enables you to 'send' a Reiki treatment to anyone, anywhere, with the same effectiveness as if that person was with you. This is sometimes referred to as practitioner level, although it is possible to practise Reiki professionally at First Degree level.

- The Third Degree is the level of a Reiki Master (Teacher), and involves essentially making a life-long commitment to the mastery of Reiki, which requires a lot of personal and spiritual development and learning, in addition to working with Reiki every day. Reiki Master training can be a short course, or it may be an apprenticeship over a longer period of time with an experienced Master. At this level you learn another symbol and mantra, some advanced healing techniques and how to attune others to the Reiki energy.

In the rest of this book you will find many techniques that will help you to 'live the Reiki way', but I should point out that if you haven't yet undertaken at least a Reiki First Degree (Reiki 1) course, you won't be able to carry out any of the Reiki techniques, as you won't yet have established a flow of the Reiki energy, which can only be acquired by receiving a Reiki attunement from a qualified Reiki Master. However, the other self-help methods that are described in the following chapters are open to anyone, whether you have learned about Reiki or not, so I hope you will give them a try.

The next chapter details the Reiki Principles that Dr Usui passed on to his students to help them to live a good life, which are the major focus of this book: just for today, don't get angry, don't worry, be grateful, work hard and be kind to others.

chapter two

THE ORIGINS OF THE REIKI PRINCIPLES

The Reiki Principles are a set of guidelines for living a fulfilled life. They were probably originally written by Emperor Mutsuhito of Japan during the Meiji period (1868–1912), and were then adopted – and possibly adapted – by Dr Mikao Usui (1865–1926), the founder of the Usui Reiki Ryoho (Usui Spiritual Energy Healing Method), a holistic healing system that originated in Japan, but which is now in use all over the world.

There are a number of translations of the Principles, but my favourite is: just for today, don't get angry, don't worry, be grateful, work hard and be kind to others.

WHICH SET OF PRINCIPLES?

You may have first come into contact with the Reiki Principles, sometimes called the Reiki Ideals, when you attended your Reiki First Degree course, or on a website or in a book about Reiki. You may have been confused because you came across different versions of the Principles, although they all still seemed pretty similar.

The wording you learn or read depends on how particular Reiki Masters were taught. For example, when I did the first level of Reiki training in 1991 I was taught the following:

1. Just for today, do not anger.
2. Just for today, do not worry.
3. Honour your parents, teachers and elders.
4. Earn your living honestly.
5. Show gratitude to every living thing.

Another form of the Reiki Principles was also in common use in the 1980s and '90s:

1. Just for today I will let go of anger.
2. Just for today I will let go of worry.
3. Today I will count my many blessings.
4. Today I will do my work honestly.
5. Today I will be kind to every living creature.

These two versions were taught by two different branches of Reiki, the first by Reiki Masters who joined the Reiki Alliance, an organization formed in 1982 under the direction of Mrs Takata's granddaughter, Phyllis Lei Furumoto, and the second by Radiance Technique Reiki Masters under the direction of Dr Barbara Ray, another of the 22 Reiki Masters taught by Mrs Takata; there may well have been other slightly different versions around at the time. However, in the late 1990s the author and Reiki Master Frank Arjava Petter, who was living and working in Japan at the time, gave us access to the original version from a document written in Dr Usui's own hand, which he translated with the help of his Japanese wife, Chetna Kobayashi, like this:

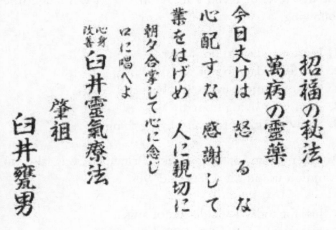

(Japanese is read from right to left)

JAPANESE	ENGLISH TRANSLATION
Shoufuku no hihoo	The secret method of inviting happiness
Manbyo no ley-yaku	The wonderful medicine for all diseases (of the body and the soul)
Kyo dake wa	Just today
1 Okoru-na	1 Don't get angry
2 Shimpai suna	2 Don't worry
3 Kansha shite	3 Be grateful (or show appreciation)

4 Goo hage me	4 Work hard (on yourself)
5 Hito ni shinsetsu ni	5 Be kind to others
Asa yuu gassho shite, koko-ro ni nenji, Kuchi ni tonaeyo	Mornings and evenings, sit in the gassho* position and repeat these words out loud and in your heart
Shin shin kaizen, Usui Reiki Ryoho	(For the) improvement of body and soul, Usui Spiritual Energy Healing Method
Chosso Usui Mikao	The founder, Mikao Usui

*Gassho means to sit quietly with your hands together in the prayer position, with your thumbs pointing to the centre of your chest, as in the illustration below.

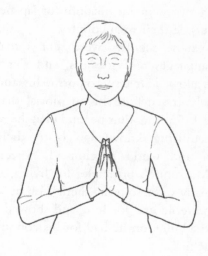

These Principles also appear on Mikao Usui's memorial, a large inscribed monolith erected in 1927 next to his grave in the public cemetery at the Saihôji Temple in the Suginami Ko district of Tokyo. There they are described as the five principles of the Meiji Emperor (Emperor Mutsuhito).

The Meiji Emperor came to the throne in Japan when Usui was only three years old, and as Usui grew up he was undoubtedly influenced by the expansiveness that was characteristic of the reign of this progressive emperor. During the Meiji Restoration period between 1868 and 1912, a new wave of openness began, as Japan's previously closed borders were opened for the first time in many centuries. Japan went from an agrarian economy to an industrial one during that time, and this resulted in an eagerness to explore the benefits of Western influences, with a consequent freedom for Japanese nationals to travel outside their own country.

Many Japanese scholars were sent abroad to study Western languages and sciences, and this relaxing of restrictions allowed Dr Usui to pursue his studies by travelling widely. It states on his memorial that he visited China, the USA and Europe, and that he was fond of reading, acquiring knowledge of medicine, history, psychology and world religions. I expect Usui had absorbed Mutsuhito's principles for living, and lived by them for many years, so using them with his students was probably quite natural for him, and showed the level of respect and admiration he had for his country's emperor and his teachings.

Perhaps it isn't surprising that in the West our form of the Principles isn't exactly the same as the recently revealed version from Japan. Mrs Takata was taught Reiki in the late 1930s, and taught it herself for over 40 years as an oral tradition, so perhaps the wording changed slightly over all that time. Or maybe the way she was taught by Hayashi wasn't quite the same. Or perhaps some of the Masters she taught didn't remember it accurately. The reason doesn't really matter, because there are great similarities between all of the versions, although the second of the Western versions seems a bit closer to the original. It is a bit of a challenge, though, to see where the Principle 'honour your parents, teachers and elders' has come from, yet it is probably just another way of interpreting 'be kind to others'. Moreover, although it may sound like it, I don't think it was ever meant to suggest that you should only be kind to older people! It's really about honouring and respecting everyone we meet for the part they play in our lives – parents, siblings, partners, friends, neighbours, colleagues, children, shop assistants, bus drivers, and so on. Also, of course, if you honour (or are kind to) others, and treat them well, they will honour and respect you. What goes around, comes around.

LIVING WITH THE REIKI PRINCIPLES TODAY

Although Dr Usui asked his students to live by the Principles in the early part of the 20th century, they are just as relevant to Reiki students – and others – today. Working more closely with the Reiki Principles is a valuable part of Reiki practice, and as you gradually absorb them into your everyday life and make them a part of you, you will inevitably find that you develop a deeper understanding of their meanings, and this is one of the purposes of this book. Here are some ideas to get you started, which are developed much further in later chapters.

Today, do not anger

Anger is usually tied to responses in the past that are of little use to us as we grow personally and spiritually, and it is generally triggered when someone or something fails to meet our expectations – or sometimes, even more importantly, when we don't come up to our own expectations. However, although it may feel uncomfortable to realize it, anger is a conscious choice, and is often just a habitual reaction to a given set of circumstances, so we *can* choose not to be angry – just for today!

Today, do not worry

In the same way we can choose not to worry. Worry is linked to our fear of the future and the unknown, and our lack of self-belief that we can cope, and it often centres around a 'what if?' scenario – a future event that is unrealized and possibly never will be. Worrying can also be a habit we get into, but it is inappropriate for people who are 'living in the moment', so we *can* choose not to worry – just for today!

Be grateful

It is important to value and appreciate many things in our lives and to be grateful for our many blessings – to develop an 'attitude of gratitude', rather than just taking things for granted, or thinking with regret about what we haven't got. Reiki is a consciousness-raising tool (as a high spiritual energy it raises our vibrations), and as our consciousness is raised, we know instinctively that every living thing is a part of us, and we are a part of it, and everything is a part of the Divine, God, the Source or whatever we choose to call it. It is therefore right to give thanks for everyone and everything in this wonderful world.

Devote yourself to your work

We need to respect whatever 'job' we have chosen for ourselves, and to honour ourselves by doing our best to create a feeling of satisfaction in that work. *All* work is valuable to the extent that we choose to value it. Also, Dr Usui's intention with Reiki was that it should be a tool for spiritual growth, so this Principle is about working towards personal growth and spiritual development each day with Reiki, and perhaps also with meditation, energy cleansing, reading self-help books, and so on. Remember that *you* are your life's work!

Be kind to others

This is about being kind to everyone we meet, under any circumstances. We make conscious choices when we make contact with people, choosing those from whom we wish to learn, those we want as friends, those we work with. But we need to honour and respect *all* the people we interact with in our lives, not just those in our inner circle, because everyone we meet is in some way one of our teachers, whether we love them or loathe them, because they are all helping us to learn and grow spiritually. We also need to extend this kindness to ourselves, because we are important, too. I am also sure this Principle is encouraging us to be kind to every living thing – animals, birds, fish and other creatures, and even to plants and the planet itself.

CHANTING THE PRINCIPLES

What Usui advised his students to do was to place their hands in gassho – palms together, fingers pointing upwards, hands held at mid-chest height – and repeat the Principles twice a day, once in the morning and once in the evening, as part of their spiritual practice, and of course you can do the same thing. You can choose the version you were taught, or the one you like best from those given above, or say the Principles in Japanese. They have a mantra-like quality when you do this, and I find I go into a beautifully quiet, meditative state after repeating them a few times, so perhaps you would like to try this. You might like to have a go at the phonetic pronunciation I've given below. It's unlikely to make you sound really Japanese, as this language is quite complex in its stresses and intonations, and of course the phonetics I have used are based on English sounds, but have a go anyway. It's only for your own satisfaction, and it can be fun.

Kyo dake wa	Kee oh dah kay wah
Okoru-na	Oh koh roo nah
Shimpai suna	Shin pie soo nah
Kansha shite	Kan shah shtay
Goo hage me	Go oh hah gay may
Hito ni shinsetsu ni	Hee toe nee shin set soo nee

In the next section I look at the first part of the Reiki Principles – 'just for today', which is about living in the moment, and the art of mindfulness and meditation.

part two

LIVING IN THE 'NOW'

Yesterday is but today's memory,
and tomorrow is today's dream.
                    Kahlil Gibran

chapter three

JUST FOR TODAY

I want to emphasize in this chapter that one of the most important aspects of the Reiki Principles is the phrase 'just for today'. This is notable for several reasons. Firstly, if you were to promise yourself, when repeating the Principles, that you would never again be angry, or never again worry, or always and forever be kind to others – well, that's a pretty tall order, and quite hard to live up to. We are all human, with all the human failings and foibles, so it's unlikely that any of us can keep permanently to the spirit of the Principles, at least at first. Making a promise to ourselves that we won't get angry today, or won't worry today, means we only have to try one day at a time, which is an achievable goal. If on occasion we don't quite manage to live up to the Principles, well, tomorrow is another day, so we can just start again – one day at a time.

The other reason why the words 'just for today' are important is that they highlight the need to live in the moment and be aware of what is going on around you; to live in the present, in the now. One of my favourite phrases is:

Yesterday is history;
Tomorrow is a mystery;

Today is a gift,
That's why it's called the present!

Most people spend the majority of their time with their minds somewhere else. Their thoughts are perpetually on what happened an hour ago, or yesterday, or last week or last year: what they wish they had said to their partner last night; why they didn't buy that bargain-price TV when they had the chance; whether they left some essential paperwork at home – and so on. Or their thoughts are constantly on what might be in the future: what's in the freezer that they can cook for dinner tonight; where to go on holiday; how to get their child to swimming practice in time; how they are going to get the money together to pay that bill, etc. Then there are always the 'what if?' scenarios to fill the mind – What if I mess up? What if I lose this job? What if my partner fancies someone else? Or even bigger things, like: If there's a recession, how will we cope? What if our house burns down or is flooded? What if I catch some awful disease? While such thoughts are spinning through your mind, you are not living life as it really is – you're on auto-pilot.

Eckhart Tolle, in his book *The Power of Now*, states 'Wherever you are, be there totally.' He suggests that some people try to escape the present with thoughts of the future and memories of the past because their 'here' is never good enough. His suggestion is that if you find your 'here and now' intolerable and it makes you unhappy, you basically have only three options:

◆ Remove yourself from the situation.

- ◆ Change the situation.
- ◆ Accept the situation totally.

A fairly stark response, maybe, but it is about taking responsibility for your life and accepting the consequences. Choose one of those options, and choose it now, is his proposition. And then get on with living, *in the present*.

TAKING TIME TO BE IN THE 'NOW'

There are some simple things you can do to practise 'being in the now'. Try this on a day when you have some time to yourself.

Use an alarm clock or cooking timer or something similar, and set it to go off once every hour for eight hours. Then when it rings, pause for 3–5 minutes, and practise being fully aware, using all your senses:

- ◆ Look around you, noticing colours, shapes, light and shadow.
- ◆ Listen to any sounds and notice their effects on you.
- ◆ Touch things around you, noticing different textures and temperatures.
- ◆ Really breathe in the scents and smells around you.
- ◆ If the alarm goes off while you're eating or drinking, really allow yourself to appreciate the taste and texture of whatever is in your mouth.

This may seem to be a very simple exercise, and you may question why you need to do it more than once a day, but it can be profound to do it every hour, because you become more sensitive to the various sensations as the day progresses. It's a good thing to repeat when life isn't going too well, or when you know you've been rushing around for days on end, because it brings things to a full stop. And it helps you to remember that you are a human *being*, not a human *doing*!

BEING PRESENT

The present moment is the one you are living now, the only moment over which you have any control, so to be present is to be alive, right now, this very minute. You may already have experienced moments of total presence, in sports or creative activities, perhaps, or when reading a good book, when the boundary between yourself and your thinking and feeling processes has dissolved or disappeared. You are completely absorbed in what you are doing at that moment in time, so you are not *doing*, but *being*. This state has been described at various times as:

- Being in the zone
- Peak experience
- Going with the flow

There isn't really any new or special technique you need to learn to be mindful, or in other words live in the 'now', in your daily life, as it is part of what happens when you concentrate fully on what is happening to you at that moment. Moreover, even though our minds are often flitting between the past and future, we do usually have some lucid moments of being totally in the present, especially if we begin to meditate, and meditation and mindfulness is discussed more fully in the next chapter.

chapter four

MINDFULNESS AND MEDITATION

Mindfulness is a Buddhist precept, meaning having your mind right here, right now, and not allowing your thoughts to wander into memories of time gone by or imaginings of time to come.

MINDFULNESS – MEDITATION IN ACTION

Part of what Dr Usui asked us to do was to be mindful and live in the present (just today) and to work hard on ourselves, by which I believe he meant working on our personal growth and spiritual development through meditation, such as the Reiki meditation and cleansing technique called Hatsurei-ho (see Chapter 15). However, the ideal of meditation practice is to be aware in every moment of your waking life, not just in those moments when you are sitting quietly, deliberately meditating. There is no more joyful place in the world than exactly where you are, right now – because you cannot experience real joy when your mind is elsewhere, thinking of what has happened in the past, or what might happen in the future.

It is possible to turn even the most mundane and potentially boring tasks into a form of meditation, to experience them fully and to learn to wonder at that experience. Try it with the washing-up. You can really experience washing-up in a completely new way if you pay real attention to it, instead of letting your mind wander, which is probably what you normally do.

- Pay attention to the feeling of the warm water on your skin.
- Pay attention to the rainbow colours in the bubbles.
- Pay attention to the rhythmic movement of your hand as it cleans a plate.
- Pay attention to the slight, squeaky sounds, as the plate becomes clean.
- Pay attention to the sparkle as you place the plate to drain.
- ... and so on.

I'm not suggesting that you slow down your washing-up to this pace every time you do it, but it's an interesting experiment, so do have a go, because it can be really valuable to take time over everyday tasks. Being more in touch with your experiences helps you to realize that you are *living*, rather than just *existing*, and that is part of the benefit of meditation.

This doesn't mean that you should perform common meditative practices all the time, such as shutting your eyes and counting your breaths while driving (please don't!), or sitting in a half-lotus position and starting to chant 'om' in the middle of the office! It does mean, however, that the awareness you develop in your daily meditation practice can naturally expand to encompass your day. It just takes a bit of practice, and it makes life much more fun because you begin to notice things that have passed you by before. You will start to see and sense more beauty around you, like the way the sun catches the edge of a cloud, or the way a smile lights up someone's face, or the softness of rain against your skin or the smell of honeysuckle.

MINDFUL LIVING

Being mindful means staying in touch with everything that is going on with us on a physical, emotional, psychological or spiritual level. Our bodies are perhaps the best benchmark we have for developing mindfulness in daily life, but most of us are not very aware of our bodies. Try the following exercise.

BEING IN TOUCH WITH YOUR BODY

Right at this moment, as you are reading this, become really aware of your body. Take an inventory.

- How are you holding your head? Is it straight up, or leaning to the left or right?
- Is your mouth relaxed, or are your lips stretched in a tense line, or slightly curved in a smile?
- Are your shoulders slightly hunched, or are you sitting straight up? If you are sitting very straight, allow your shoulders and body to relax, and see if that

feels different. If you're hunched over a little, sit up really straight, and see how your body feels like that.

- Maybe some parts of your body are feeling warm, while others feel cold? Perhaps you can feel a draught?
- Sense the chair beneath you.
- Sense your feet on the floor.
- Become aware of where your hands are – perhaps resting on your lap, or on the arm of the chair.
- Feel the breath being drawn in through your nose and hear the sound it makes.
- Hear the other sounds in the room. Maybe you can hear other people breathing? Perhaps you can hear traffic noise outside, or someone playing a musical instrument, or the hum of conversation from a nearby TV or radio, or the clattering of dishes in the kitchen?
- Now that you've become more aware of your surroundings, let yourself move into a few minutes of sitting quietly, just concentrating on your breathing, letting your breaths become slow and deep. Let each in-breath become slightly slower, deeper and longer.
- Let there be a pause before you breathe out again, and let the air out slowly, until you're sure your lungs are really empty. Then let there be another pause, before you breathe in again.
- As you adopt this slow, calm breathing, notice how your body begins to feel more relaxed. Perhaps you can sense your heart rate slowing down, too.

You may not realize it, but this is a fairly classic method of meditation – becoming fully aware of something, or in other words, being mindful. Continue the exercise in silence for a while – for as long or as short a time as you feel comfortable. It could be just 2–3 minutes, or 10–20 minutes, or half an hour. Choose what feels right for you.

WHY MEDITATE?

Meditation is really a holistic discipline. It creates change at all levels of being, including the physical, emotional and psychological. It also has the power to awaken us to the spiritual levels of our being, and enables us to discover who we really are and what we might achieve. It brings us to a state of self-realization that is the highest expression of the human nature.

Why do people meditate? What would be *your* main reason to meditate? Would it be for improved health, relaxation, stress prevention or reduction, self-realization or spiritual inspiration? Hopefully this chapter will give you various ideas that will help you to choose the most appropriate way for you to meditate, and will take away some of the myths about meditation that tend to frighten people off, or make them believe they can't do it. First let's look at what meditation is, and what methods are available to us.

What is Meditation?

Meditation is an umbrella word that encompasses a multitude of techniques aimed at achieving an altered state of consciousness, resulting in a deeply relaxed state that can eventually bring about a state of enlightenment or ecstasy or both. There are two major types of meditation.

1. Most Christian, Sufi and yoga meditation techniques are based on heightened concentration, where you give your undivided attention to a single idea or perception, seeking the total absorption that leads to understanding. If this is successful it leads to a trance-like state where external awareness dims and the effects of competing external stimuli fade away. This is probably the oldest type of meditation, and it is found in most cultures in some form.

2. The other type of meditation is Buddhist, which is itself divided into two strands – samatha, which means calm, and vipassana, which means insight. Both involve the passive examination, and then letting go, of whatever content drifts into the individual's awareness. Samatha is designed to bring peaceful awareness and acceptance, and vipassana to bring mindfulness and understanding.

That may make it sound quite difficult, but it doesn't have to be. The myth about meditation is that you have to completely empty your mind, preferably while sitting in the lotus position – and if that's your starting point then it's no wonder people give up quite quickly! Certainly, the aim is to quieten the mind, but to totally empty it is probably only possible for those with many years of practice. It is estimated that we have at least 60,000 thoughts each day, and our minds are busy even when we're asleep, so achieving a quieter, more peaceful state is all you really need to aim for. You can start with just a few minutes, and gradually build up the time you spend in meditation. Don't jump straight in and aim for half an hour, because you will probably feel frustrated and uncomfortable, start fidgeting and give up the whole process. Try five minutes – or even 2–3 – to start with.

My view is that meditation allows you to experience and enjoy a feeling of being at one with yourself and with the Universe. It brings an acceptance of yourself and your part in 'the grand scheme of things', and leads to a deepening of 'inner knowing', as opposed to simply having acquired knowledge. Meditation is a mental and spiritual discipline that is open to anyone who is willing to try it. Successful meditation does require some practice and self-discipline, but after a while you will find it quite easy, and it will become a natural part of daily life.

In all forms of meditation, therefore, there is a focus and a quietening of the mind. This aims at first simply to reduce, and eventually to eliminate, the chatter of daily life, the stresses of the environment in which we live, and so provide a haven within which we are free to connect with our inner being. It helps us to overcome the problems and illusions we create for ourselves and that we allow others to create for us, and also to overcome habits we have formed that hold us back. Meditation allows us to go beyond the everyday, into who we really are. The art of focusing, and awareness of being in the moment, changes brain activity, which leads to a psychological opening up of ourselves to compassion, joy, contentment and fulfilment.

The Physiological Effects of Meditation

Lots of research has been done into the effects of meditation on the body, particularly on the activity of the brain, nervous system and immune system. As mentioned, meditation is an altered state of consciousness, and some researchers have suggested that there are various stages of consciousness, from deep sleep to highly active wakefulness. Various brain activities can be measured, and tracing these patterns has produced waves of different frequencies:

- Beta waves, (the highest frequency), associated with active wakefulness.
- Alpha waves, associated with relaxed wakefulness.
- Theta waves, associated with dreaming.
- Delta waves (the lowest frequency), associated with sleep.

Meditation has been shown to increase alpha–wave activity, which has led to the suggestion that it acts as a form of self-hypnosis and relaxation. The alterations in brain activity caused by meditation apparently have profound effects on the autonomic nervous system – the part of the nervous system that controls digestion, breathing, heart rate and blood pressure, and that enables our body to respond to everyday stresses. It appears that, particularly with the increase in alpha waves produced by some forms of meditation, the autonomic nervous system responds by reducing activity in the 'fight, flight and freeze' responses, reducing heart rate and blood pressure, calming the breathing and thus generally reducing the stress on the body.

A relatively new topic for research is in the area of psycho-neuro immunology, which examines the effect of the mind on the nervous system and immune systems. Again, there is the suggestion that meditation reduces the stresses on the immune system, thus allowing the body to defend itself more easily against infection, and to promote healing by responding to, and overcoming, invading micro-organisms and cancerous and other rogue cells.

Meditation is therefore seen by many health professionals to be an aid to stress reduction, to have beneficial effects on the body and to promote good health in general.

Methods of Meditation

A variety of methods can be used for meditation:

- Chanting or singing, using repeated simple phrases or mantras.
- Transcendental Meditation (going beyond the individual).
- Seeking the 'great void' or Nirvana (as in Buddhism).
- Meditation on objects, such as feathers or stones.
- Meditation on symbols, such as icons or mandalas.
- Meditation on a flame, such as a candle flame.
- Meditation on nature – trees, plants, water or a landscape.
- Meditation on the four elements – earth, air, fire and water (this occurs in both Eastern and Western spiritual traditions).

◆ Meditation with sound, such as Tibetan gongs or the sounds of nature.

◆ Meditation on colour.

◆ Meditation on qualities – loving kindness, compassion, happiness and joy.

◆ Meditation on the body and its natural activities – breathing, walking, moving and resting.

◆ Guided meditation, usually called visualization, which takes you on an inner journey to your deeper self.

All methods of meditation are equally valid, so you might want to try out quite a few in your search for the technique that fits you best, or you may find that using a combination of meditation forms is the way for you to develop. Later in this chapter there are examples of several types of meditation for you to try.

Preparing to Meditate

Anyone can learn to meditate, but there are some things that make it easier and more effective. Meditation does require a level of self-discipline, and in terms of producing permanent changes and helping with your spiritual journey of personal growth and development, regular meditation is seen as an essential practice. By all means start off with just a few minutes a day to help you develop the habit of regular meditation, but you should ideally aim after a while to do at least 20 minutes a day.

When meditating you will need to be in a safe, quiet environment, one in which you feel comfortable and where you will either be undisturbed, or where disturbances will be as few as is possible, although when you are more experienced you will find you can enter a meditation state almost anywhere, regardless of the noises around you – a railway station, a busy park or while sitting with a coffee in a café.

Bright light stimulates the body and can make meditation more difficult, whereas complete darkness tends to promote sleep, so soft lighting, such as candlelight, is usually best, and many people find candles with their flickering flames to be an aid to meditation in their own right. Some people like to burn incense or essential oils such as lavender, or a scented candle, and you will need to ensure that the room is at an appropriate temperature – too cold and it will prevent concentration, too warm and it is likely to make you sleepy. It is also a good idea to remove glasses, large pieces of jewellery and your watch, and some people like to remove their shoes as well.

Posture is important, as having a straight back will help your inner energies to flow better, and this is best accomplished sitting in a supportive chair or on a cushion on the floor with your back against a wall, with your hands loosely relaxed in your lap or resting on your knees, or in a classic prayer position (although this can be a bit tiring after a while). Of course, it is possible to meditate while lying on the floor or on a bed, but this often induces sleep. Crossing the legs or arms can make meditation more difficult unless you can assume a completely cross-legged posture such as the lotus position, which if you are agile enough is a very satisfying position in which to meditate – but don't force the issue. Only try this if you feel reasonably comfortable.

It can be very helpful to establish a meditation routine, by meditating for a certain length of time at a particular time of day. Some people find meditation best in the early morning, while others prefer to meditate during the evening, so choose a time that's convenient for you. Bear in mind that it is difficult to enter a proper meditative state after a heavy meal, and even more so after drinking alcohol, so it is best to wait at least two hours after eating, or to meditate beforehand, otherwise you may become too sleepy.

Meditation on the Breath

Perhaps the easiest and best way to begin meditation is with the breath. Breathing is essential to life. We start our lives with an in-breath, and end them with an out-breath, and breathing is something that we mostly take for granted, unless we are unfortunate enough to have an illness or some other reason that causes breathing difficulties. Yet it is really a miraculous process, which continues thousands of times a day without any conscious effort or control from us.

- To begin with, close your eyes and concentrate on your breathing.
- Let your breathing become slower and deeper, allowing the breath to be inhaled to its fullest extent, and allowing it to be exhaled completely.
- Try to be aware of where the air is going, how far down your chest it is travelling. Perhaps place a hand on your chest and feel it rising up and down.
- Place a hand on your solar plexus (your midriff), and feel it going up and down.
- Move your hand down to your abdomen. Is it also

going up and down? Can you deepen your breathing to make your abdomen move?

◆ Start to count your breaths, counting each in-breath until you reach the number nine. Then start again at one, and just enjoy some silent meditation for a few minutes, continuing to concentrate and counting your breaths from one to nine for as long as you feel comfortable.

The Four-fold Breath

This is a slightly different form of breathing meditation, where the in-breath, out-breath and the spaces between breaths are given equal time.

◆ Breathe in with a deep but comfortable breath from the diaphragm to the count of four (about four seconds).

◆ Hold your breath for the count of four.

◆ Breathe out slowly to the count of four.

◆ Hold the lungs empty to the count of four.

◆ Start again.

This exercise has a very relaxing effect on the body, and when you are quite practised you will find that you can increase the length of time for each stage to five, six or seven seconds, although I wouldn't advise lengthening it beyond about nine seconds, as it then becomes more a state of endurance than a state of meditation.

Meditation Using Mantras

A mantra is a sound, phrase or prayer that is repeated over and over again, either aloud (spoken or sung) or as a thought, which is believed to bring meditational benefits to the person chanting it. You may have heard of people chanting 'om', which is a Sanskrit mantra that might also be incorporated into a phrase such as 'om ah hum', where 'om' represents the body, 'ah' the speech and 'hum' the mind. The chanting of these words is believed to be a prayer that purifies negativity produced by the body, speech and thought, as well as bringing a blessing to the person chanting it.

♦ Sit in a comfortable posture with your eyes closed.

♦ Bring the mantra 'om ah hum' (or another phrase or word you have chosen, such as 'love and compassion') into your consciousness, and begin repeating it slowly, either silently in your mind, or aloud, speaking as distinctly as possible. (If you wish, you can use musical tones for chanting, singing rather than speaking, either the same note three times, i.e. once each for 'om', 'ah' and 'hum', or three different notes.) You may feel the need to gradually increase the speed of repetitions – or not. If you are chanting aloud you may run out of breath, but this is quite natural. Just breathe deeply for a few moments, then continue with the chant.

♦ Stop whenever you need to. With practice you will find it easier to incorporate your inhalations and exhalations with the repetitions of the mantra, but there is no need to try too hard; just let it happen naturally. As you recite the mantra you may find that you naturally relax into the sound, your breath and your attention combining effortlessly and powerfully.

- Repeat the mantra for three, five, seven, nine or eleven minutes – whichever feels best to you. (I would suggest three minutes to start with, until you're more practised at this technique.)

- As you reach the end of your mantra meditation period, it is good practice to gently slow down the repetitions, rather than coming to an abrupt stop.

- When you've finished, sit quietly and explore your awareness. Take note of the feelings in your body and mind. You might feel relaxed and at peace, receive an insight into some area of your life, experience colours in your inner vision or sense that some form of cleansing or healing has taken place.

Meditation on Sound

People react to sounds in very different ways. For example, some people enjoy listening to loud rock or pop music with a strong beat, while others prefer classical music, jazz or folk music. For meditation purposes, rock, pop, jazz and folk are probably not the best inspirations, as they are rarely calming and relaxing, but some people enjoy listening to classical or 'New Age' music playing in the background as they meditate.

Traditional sounds for meditation include Tibetan bowls made of seven different metals, which have a special resonance depending upon their size; or ting-shah, which are pairs of small, flat, cymbal-shaped pieces of metal, usually joined together on either end of a piece of thin leather or cord, or Tibetan gongs that can vary in size from about 12 in (30 cm) to 48 in (122 cm) in diameter. Other sounds that encourage meditation are recordings (or live performances) of monks chanting, or soft, rhythmic drumming, such as a combination of three-beat, five-beat and seven-beat drumming in the Celtic tradition.

There are plenty of CDs on the market, from Tibetan monks chanting 'om' and chanting special rhythms to link to each of the seven chakras, to Native American drumming and 'New Age' music from flutes and guitars, to whale song and other natural sounds, so this might be something you would like to try. Some of my favourite titles are given on page 255.

A Relaxation Practice

Two great tools to aid meditation are relaxation and breathing control, and as part of the process of meditation you may wish to develop the habit of relaxing your body by visualizing and feeling it relax.

- ◆ Sit in a comfortable position.
- ◆ Feel your feet on the floor, then tense the muscles of your toes, feet and heels, and relax them completely.
- ◆ Tense the muscles of your calves, knees and thighs, then let them relax.
- ◆ Tense the muscles of your hips, abdomen and

chest, and let them relax, then slow your breathing to an even rate.

◆ Tense, then relax the muscles in your shoulders, arms, hands and fingers.

◆ Tense, then relax the muscles in your neck, jaw, face and scalp.

This method is useful because we tend to store a lot of tension in our muscles, particularly in our shoulders and legs, so you might like to tense and relax those areas 3–4 times. When you're feeling relaxed – with practice this will only take 2–3 minutes – become aware of your breathing, and perhaps count the breaths. Allow yourself to fall into a slow, regular pattern of breathing – then you can choose which method of meditation to use.

Dealing with Distractions

One of the major problems encountered in meditation is difficulty in getting rid of the thoughts, sounds and activities of daily life. However, if you try too hard, concentrating on getting rid of these distractions, you will actually make it more difficult for yourself, because you will generate even more thoughts. If you work on the principle that all our thoughts and activities are worthy of acknowledgement, just acknowledge them, then let them go.

There are many techniques for letting go, and here are three for you to try:

1. If a thought, or recognition of a sound such as a car, or the humming of central heating, comes into your mind, try to visualize that thought or sound, and surround it with a bubble of light, or a balloon, then watch it float up and up and out of your mind.

2. You may see thoughts as birds flying across the sky. Acknowledge their presence. Visualize each thought or noise as a bird, then allow it to fly away, out of the scene in your mind.

3. Some people like to visualize intruding thoughts in a candle flame. They may float up with the heat and smoke of the candle, or the thought may be imagined within the flame and the candle snuffed out. The candle can always be relit (in your imagination) should another intruding thought drift by.

There may be occasions when you want to remember a thought for later use. In this case you could visualize a box or basket into which the thought bubble can be placed, then the lid can be put on the box to hold the bubble inside until later. Such thoughts can be retrieved after the meditation has finished, if you wish.

WHAT IS VISUALIZATION?

Visualization, sometimes called guided meditation, is a method of meditation in which your soul or spirit, sometimes called your 'Higher Self', allows images to develop within the mind. These images can be symbols, objects, landscapes, people, animals, plants or colours, which may be familiar or new to you. Although these images may initially seem to be unrelated, they will often form a story, which may be allegorical, or more directly understandable as an exploration of your personal truth, the knowledge and insight you are seeking, an understanding of your desires and needs, or a spiritual awareness of some kind.

Visualizations can have a variety of purposes – they can be used for self-development, healing, relaxation, relieving stress or seeking greater union with the Divine/Source/Universe. They are also often good fun!

In visualizations you allow your soul or spirit to influence your mind and present you with new ideas, or maybe a different way of looking at things. Often some natural object, or a word someone says, allows our mind to go somewhere else, a state we might describe as 'daydreaming', which is usually a pleasant and occasionally helpful activity. Visualization is a much more structured, supportive and effective vehicle for doing this.

When you begin visualizations you may see only part of an image, or you may see an image for only a few moments. 'Seeing' may seem more 'knowing' what is there, or imagining what is there, or a feeling, or it may even appear in words. All of these 'sensings' are valid parts of visualization, and the more often you take yourself on visual inner journeys, the more the focus of what you 'see' will become clearer, more defined and more definite. Thus your visualizing will potentially begin to lead you and expand you out of a set visualization, and bring you deeper and broader understanding.

One problem with visualization is that some people believe they can't do it, and this is usually because they have unrealistic expectations of what they should 'see'.

Granted, some people are very visual, and do see things very clearly in their visualizations, but others do not.

♦ Try this. Can you remember, by 'seeing' it in your mind, what your bedroom looks like? In your imagination, can you 'move' around the room and see it from different angles? That's the type of image you might have when you are visualizing.

♦ Try something else. Here's a short list of things that will probably trigger visual images in your mind: elephant, cat, tree, flower. The way you see each of these things might be different from the way others see it – for instance, you might see a black cat, while someone else might see a ginger cat; you might see a rose, but another person may see a daffodil. That's quite natural, because the images which come to mind are usually familiar ones, so you will 'see' something you know.

♦ The same is true, initially, if you visualize a landscape. You will probably see a countryside, seaside or woodland scene that you have seen in real life. However, after a bit of practice your mind will present you with 'new' landscapes that are no less real to you, but which exist only as imaginings – and that can be quite exciting!

The Visualization Process
In this book there are a number of visualizations that are obviously given in print, and it is useful to read each one through 2–3 times before you start, to enable you to become familiar with its pattern. Alternatively you might choose to let someone read it out to you slowly, or you could prepare a CD for yourself so that you can play it back whenever you wish. Eventually you can try creating

your own visualizations – if you do so, be clear what you want to focus on, or what question you want answered, before you start.

Initially try to follow each visualization the way it is set out, but if your soul or spirit directs you to a different place or different things, or if within your visualization someone comes to greet you, that is what you need at that time, and you should go along with the new 'route'. However, if you're following your own visualization, try not to let it continue too long, because the benefit lies in taking note of the emotions and the knowledge that it brings – it isn't a good idea to overload yourself with detail, especially when you're just beginning to visualize on a regular basis. It is also very important, if you're following your own visualization, to always bring yourself back to the point where you started the visualization (i.e. the first scene you imagined) before your awareness fully returns to the room you are in.

After a Visualization

At the end of a visualization, give yourself a minute or two to become aware of your surroundings once again, and when you are ready, open your eyes. It is helpful to note down straight away as much as you can remember of the visualization, so keep a notebook and pen nearby. Don't worry if at first you don't see much detail, or you don't remember very much. You can always return to the visualization at another time, and, indeed, repeat it again and again if you want to, and gradually the fuller picture will develop.

One idea you could try is to do the same visualization every day for a week, then collate a list of the symbols and gifts to explore in meditation over the following week. For this you will need to keep a journal or diary of your visualizations to record what you experience – this can be a very helpful document in its own right, especially when you look back in it from some time in the future, as it can be a record of your spiritual progress and personal growth.

Feeling Safe When Visualizing

As previously mentioned, it is important to feel safe and secure when meditating, and one of the best ways of promoting a feeling of safety is by using the power of your mind to create a protective barrier of white light (or Reiki). This first visualization allows you to fill yourself with white light, bringing it down from the Divine Source into the crown of your head and moving it throughout your whole body, finally spreading the white light out around you to fill the space in which you are sitting, to provide a protective screen around you. You also anchor yourself into the earth with roots of white light, and this gives a further feeling of security. With practice, the visualization of white light becomes easier and quicker, and takes perhaps only 30 seconds or a minute. Many people like to carry out this visualization every time they meditate, as the feeling of protection allows them to relax more deeply.

BRINGING IN THE LIGHT

◆ Sit in a comfortable position and allow your body to relax. Begin to be aware of your breathing, and follow your breath in and out, in and out; with each breath you are becoming more and more relaxed.

◆ Visualize an opening at the top of your head, and see a thin thread of white light passing up through the ceiling, through the roof and up into the sky above.

◆ See this thread of light going through the edge of the Earth's atmosphere and out into space, moving further and further out until you feel it connecting with the Divine Source, a huge mass of brilliant white light, and allow that white light to flow back down the thread, making it bigger and brighter, and allow the light to flow right down into your head.

◆ The brilliant light now fills your head, and moves down into your neck, shoulders and arms, and right down into your hands to the very tips of your fingers.

◆ You see it flowing through your chest and back, and down into your abdomen and hips, and then into your thighs, knees, calves, ankles and feet, right to the tips of your toes.

◆ You feel your feet becoming heavier and more solid, feel the connection with the floor beneath you, then allow the white light to flow out of your feet into the earth.

- Imagine the white light forming roots growing from your feet down into the earth, anchoring you and making you feel very secure.
- Now the whole of your body is flooded with white light – you can use this light to form a protective barrier around you.
- Imagine that the light is coming out of your hands and visualize yourself moving your hands over all of your body so that a cloak of white light surrounds you.
- Now allow that light to spread out, filling the room to create a safe and sacred space, and watch the light swirl into all the corners, from floor to ceiling, from wall to wall, from door to window, until the whole room is bathed in white light.
- Just enjoy the peace and tranquillity of your protected space, and allow any stray thoughts that come into your mind to simply drift across. Remain in a relaxed, meditative state for five or ten minutes, or as long as you feel comfortable.

In the rest of this book we look at the Reiki Principles in more depth. In Part 3 we concentrate on the first of Dr Usui's Principles: 'just for today, do not anger'.

part three

LIVING WITHOUT ANGER

Your emotions can guide you, but you don't have to let them control you.

Penelope Quest

chapter five

UNDERSTANDING EMOTIONS

'Living without anger' is the theme of Part 3, which might seem a difficult thing to do – surely everyone feels angry sometimes? But 'just for today, do not anger' is the first of the Reiki Principles Dr Usui passed on to us, so in this and the next chapter I show you why you might get angry, what anger does to you, and how to cope with it and heal it. However, anger is only one of the many distressing emotions we experience that can potentially produce harmful reactions in us – and I feel sure that the essence of what Dr Usui was guiding us to do was to live more equably. Therefore before we look at anger specifically, in this chapter I want to explore the theory of emotions and how they can either help or hinder us in our attempt to 'live the Reiki way'.

WHAT ARE EMOTIONS?

We have over 600 words in the English language to describe emotions, and we use up to 42 muscles in our faces to express them, but the six most common emotions are happiness, sadness, surprise, disgust, fear and anger.

Emotions are thought to arise in the part of the brain known as the limbic system, which is a primitive system that also exists in all other mammals and some reptiles, and it represents a part of our survival mechanism. What was once perhaps just a mechanism that allowed us to react to danger – feelings of fear release adrenaline in our bodies to get us ready for 'fight or flight' – has evolved over millions of years into a delicate and sophisticated internal guidance system. Our emotions basically help us to:

- Identify when our basic human needs are, or are not, being met.
- Identify whether our choices or decisions 'feel' good or bad.
- Identify whether we feel safe or unsafe with someone's behaviour so that we can set comfortable boundaries.
- Provide verbal and non-verbal communication (e.g. facial expressions) to signal to others how we feel, to facilitate interpersonal interaction.
- Potentially provide a way of uniting us as a species (e.g. empathy, compassion, cooperation, forgiveness).
- Identify what makes us happy or unhappy.

So, for example, if you feel fear, you will try to escape from the danger; if you feel disgusted, you might move away from whatever makes you feel like that; if you're feeling happy, you will relax; so your emotions influence your behaviour. We use our emotions for making decisions to help us in our daily lives. For instance, when we meet people we look at their faces to assess whether we know them, to judge their gender and age, and to see what mood they are in.

Most of us are pretty good at identifying the facial expressions that indicate the six basic emotions described above – happiness, sadness, fear, anger, surprise and disgust – and we are therefore able to react appropriately.

GENERATING EMOTIONS

Emotions result when feelings are filtered through our beliefs, when we develop judgements about what we should, or should not, be feeling. So, for example, if someone in front of you jumps the queue in a shop and gets served before you, you could either accept the situation, shrug your shoulders and wait your turn, which would not generate any specific emotion or, if you were in a hurry and believed that person would make you late for something important, you might react with anger, even possibly challenging them verbally to reinstate your place in the queue. However, emotions are not caused by outer events. They are an internal reaction to an external event. They represent a choice you have made. We choose what emotion to feel. *Always.* So emotions aren't automatic reactions to situations or events; they form a part of our complex responses to life – our personalities. They are based on our life experiences so far, which is why people – each person being individual – react in diverse ways to the same situations.

EMOTIONAL PROGRAMMING

All of your experiences since you were a small child have had an impact on you, and although your emotions are always generated within you, you learn your particular range of emotions from the people who were influential in your life, especially when you were young. Effectively, you have been receiving emotional programming since you were old enough to discern facial, verbal and physical expressions, and in your early years this would have been from your parents or care-givers, siblings, teachers and friends. Scientists believe that even if you don't remember an actual emotional event from childhood, you will remember what you felt, which becomes an emotional memory that can be triggered by something you saw, heard or even smelt at the time, and those memories might still affect you as an adult.

In the modern world your emotional programming can also come from TV, films and even computer games, because these reflect images of emotions to which we are susceptible, especially when we're young. Think of the huge range of emotions, from intolerable grief to over-whelming happiness, sexual desire to violent anger, demonstrated in any of TV's soap operas, for example. It is this emotional programming that is one of the foundations for our belief system, which we integrate into our subconscious, and which then provides us with our patterns of behaviour and habitual emotional responses.

Psychological research has shown that if either or both of your parents showed little emotion, laughing or crying infrequently, and rarely or never hugging or holding you, you are likely to grow up suppressing your emotions, because you believe it is the way to be. Alternatively, you may have been exposed to a parent who was overly emotional, crying easily or losing their temper regularly, so this would be the 'norm' to you, and you are likely to follow in their footsteps. We all learn by example, and what we learn eventually becomes absorbed into our own personalities, so that pattern continues from one generation to another.

Of course, we do have other choices. Sometimes people react against their programming, and if their childhood was miserable because of harsh or restrictive and unloving parents, they will behave in the opposite way when they are adults, becoming loving, tolerant and demonstrative. But that only goes to show that our emotions, and the way we express them, are choices. Just because we have formed a subconscious habit and react to certain situations in a certain way doesn't mean we have to continue doing so for ever. We can change our reactions.

Positive and Negative

Perhaps this sounds as though having emotions is pretty undesirable? Not so. We have a huge range of emotions that we can enjoy, as well as those which aren't so much fun. Of course, extremes of emotion can cause problems. Sadness can become depression, anger can become unprovoked aggression, and pleasure can lead to addiction. Feeling afraid in a dangerous situation is natural and useful, but being too fearful can cause unhelpful anxiety, phobias and panic attacks. However, there are many more positive emotions we can choose to feel as well. How about feeling elated, ecstatic or enthralled? Or enlivened, energetic or enthusiastic?

EMOTIONS AS GUIDANCE

I've already mentioned that our emotions were originally part of our survival instinct, and that in our modern world we use them to guide us in our everyday interactions with other people. However, there is another, more innovative, metaphysical viewpoint — that emotions are actually part of our spiritual guidance system — a way in which our Soul, sometimes referred to as our Higher Self, can communicate with us.

From this perspective, if you are feeling fearful, depressed or pessimistic, this indicates that something is 'wrong' in your life, or you are not going in the 'right' direction, whereas if you are feeling enthusiastic, optimistic or content, then you are on the 'right path' — doing what you need to do, being who you really are. The most comprehensive explanation of the relationship between emotions and their effect on our lives can be found in a book I highly recommend — *Ask and It Is Given* by Esther and Jerry Hicks, who report the channelled spiritual teachings of Abraham. (Abraham is not a living person, he is a highly evolved entity — a collection of souls who may or may not have lived physical lives — who lives on the spiritual realm, whose wisdom and insight is 'channelled' through Esther Hicks, a psychic medium who lives in the USA.) I will try to explain, briefly, some of the theories described in this book.

The Emotional Hierarchy

Abraham explains that all emotions can be classified on a hierarchy from the lowest, darkest feelings such as fear, grief or despair, up to the highest, lightest feelings such as love and joy.

love, joy, enthusiasm, passion, trust, freedom, empowerment, gratitude, eagerness

happiness, optimism, contentment, hope, positive expectation

boredom, pessimism, frustration, impatience, irritation

feeling overwhelmed, disappointment, doubt, worry

blame, discouragement, anger, revenge

rage, hatred, jealousy

insecurity, guilt, lack of self-worth

fear, grief, depression,
despair,
powerlessness

At the top of the scale, when you're feeling full of love, joy and gratitude, you are said to be in alignment with who you truly are, and are fully connected with the Source (or God or the Universe). At this level your life feels good, you're having fun, with nice people around you, and you seem to attract good things to you, so you feel enthusiastic about life, and you're happy to be alive.

Down at the bottom of the scale, though, when you're consumed with grief, or full of fear, you are out of alignment with the real you, and less connected with the Source, so the people around you reflect depressing feelings and confirm your sense of powerlessness, and you feel on a never-ending spiral of despair.

MOVING UP THE EMOTIONAL SCALE

Fortunately there is a way out of that spiral of despair, but it doesn't take you straight up to the top. The way up the

63

emotional scale is usually taken one or at the most two steps at a time. Let's take one emotional example – grief – which has a classic recovery schedule that, psychologists tell us, normally takes about three years. If you're feeling in the depths of despair because you're grieving over the death of a loved one, having people tell you to cheer up, or suggest happy affirmations to 'bring you out of it', or plan fun, exciting things for you to do, is absolutely the last thing you can stand. But then you might feel guilty, because you know your friends or relatives are trying to help you, or you may even sink into feelings of unworthiness, not believing you deserve their help because you're so unwilling to accept it – but actually guilt and feelings of unworthiness are one stage up the hierarchy, so that can be a step in the right direction.

Later, as you begin to get over the shock of your loved one's death, you might react to their suggestions with rage – how dare they interfere? Why can't they leave you alone? Or you might feel rage towards the person who has died, for leaving you, but that's actually a natural reaction, and it's another step upwards on the emotional hierarchy. The next step might be to blame someone or something for your loss – perhaps the doctors who didn't save your loved one, or the driver of the car who injured them, but again, that's a very normal response, and you've stepped up the scale again.

That doesn't mean that rage and blame are good places to be, of course, but they do indicate that you are starting to engage with your situation, which is a more positive reaction than being right down in the depths of despair, where your feelings tend to overwhelm you so that you don't feel able to do anything. Although rage and blame are negative emotions, they are more active than passive, which means they are a little higher up the emotional scale – and they may also make you more likely to be a bit more receptive to positive suggestions from those who care about you. However, there's still quite a way to go before you begin to recognize that your situation has improved – and although it's a cliché, they do say that time is a great healer. You may need to work your way through some worry and doubt and frustration, perhaps wondering how you will cope without your loved one, before you can start to feel more content, hopeful or optimistic. Eventually, however, you will regain your passion and enthusiasm for life; you will feel happy and joyful, and wake up each morning eager to face a new day. It just takes some time.

The idea of a hierarchy of emotions may seem a bit complicated, but hopefully the example I've given shows that with time we can – and do – move out of depressing and negative emotions into more satisfying and enjoyable feelings. That is perhaps as far as I can go with this theory in this chapter, so if you would like to learn more about the hierarchy of emotions, do read *Ask and It Is Given*. In Part 5 I return to another aspect of Abraham's theory, about the power of thought and the Law of Attraction, so hopefully it will become a bit clearer – and you will learn how to use your thoughts and emotions to create the kind of life you want. Here I suggest a few techniques that can prove invaluable in changing your emotions for the better, and getting you up the emotional hierarchy at a much faster pace. The first two are Reiki techniques, naturally, but then I introduce you to an innovative method called Emotional Freedom Technique, or EFT, which I have found to be an effective and interesting way of dealing with negative emotions. As I mentioned in the Introduction, *Living the Reiki Way* isn't only about using Reiki – it can encompass other methods which help you to cope with overwhelming emotions or problems of any kind.

USING REIKI TO HEAL YOUR EMOTIONS

One way of carrying out emotional healing is to use Reiki, of course, and there are advantages to being able to use the Reiki symbols for this, if you have already done a Reiki Second Degree course, but if not, you can simply let the Reiki flow and it will do its job, although it may take just a little longer. In case you are not familiar with the term 'chakra', which I use in the technique below, it is a Sanskrit word meaning wheel or vortex, and is used to describe some energy centres in the body. The seven main chakras are located near the perineum (base), the navel (sacral), the midriff (solar plexus), the chest (heart), the throat (throat), the brow (third eye) and the top of the head (crown).

1. Decide which emotions you want to work on. You can work on more than one at a time, or link similar types of emotion together. You may choose to deal with fear, nervousness, depression, anger, sadness, grief, impatience, stress or any other emotion that you feel needs healing.

2. Decide where you generally feel these emotions. For example, anger, fear or problems with self-esteem are often felt in the solar plexus; loneliness, grief or rejection in the heart area; money or job worries in the base chakra; jealousy about sexual relationships in the sacral chakra, and so on.

3. Next, if you have Reiki Second Degree, draw, or imagine, a large Harmony (Mental and Emotional) symbol over what seems to be the most appropriate chakra (if you're not sure, draw the symbol over your crown chakra), then visualize the symbol expanding until it encompasses the whole of you, say its mantra three times, and ask and *intend* that it brings its gentle, healing, peaceful and restorative energy to fill your physical and energy bodies, to bring greater harmony and balance to your life, and to heal your feelings of . . . (*name whatever emotion(s) you want to work on*).

4. If you don't have Reiki Second Degree, place both your hands over the appropriate chakra, and imagine and *intend* that Reiki is flowing out of your hands, and ask and *intend* that Reiki heals, harmonizes and balances your physical and energy bodies, to bring greater harmony and balance to your life, and to heal your feelings of . . . (*name the emotion(s) you want to work on*).

5. Let yourself stay in a meditative state, giving yourself Reiki, and imagine being surrounded and encompassed by Reiki for at least 5 minutes, but preferably for about 15 minutes, until you feel much calmer and more content, then either take your hands away

and place them in the gassho (prayer) position, giving thanks to Reiki with a little bow, or if you have Reiki Second Degree, draw a Power symbol to seal in the peaceful energies, saying its mantra three times, then gassho and give thanks.

6. Finally, clap your hands or shake them vigorously to break the energy connections.

Repeat this exercise on a daily basis, working with one or more emotions, until you sense that they have changed, and feel less strong or less troublesome. A good check for this is to think of some situation that would normally trigger the type of emotion you are working on, let yourself imagine it as vividly as possible and see if you get any reaction in the appropriate chakra. If you don't, then at least some healing has occurred, but of course you can always repeat the process any time those emotions resurface – if they ever do.

A SIMPLE REIKI TECHNIQUE

If you are feeling churned up, anxious or irritated, and all you want to do is to feel calmer or more centred, then a simple way of using Reiki is to place one hand on your heart chakra (roughly over your breastbone) and the other on your solar plexus (midriff), and allow the Reiki to flow, intending that it helps you to become calm and centred. Stay like this for 5–10 minutes, or until you feel that your emotional state has become more composed.

EMOTIONAL FREEDOM TECHNIQUE (EFT)

Although my first reaction is always to turn to Reiki to help me to feel better, there are other techniques that I have found useful and would like to share with you. One of the most effective is called the Emotional Freedom Technique (EFT). This was developed by Gary Craig, based on a system of psychological healing called Thought Field Therapy (TFT), which was originally developed by a clinical psychologist, Dr Roger Callahan. He based his system on acupuncture points and kinesiology, and his most famous case was a patient called Mary who had such a severe water phobia that she couldn't go out in the rain, or even look at water on TV. Having tried everything else he could think of, he eventually tapped on her stomach meridian (the end of one of the energy lines running throughout the body, used in acupuncture, acupressure and reflexology), below the eye, and astonishingly 20 seconds later, the phobia was completely gone, and she was able to stand by a swimming pool and splash her face with water.

EFT is therefore a form of Energy Psychology that uses the energetic pathways through the body, the meridians. These relay information to the entire energy system, as well as channelling vital energy to the organs and tissues of the physical body, and the energy within each meridian also registers emotions, feelings and sensations. Each time we experience an emotion, the body's energy system is influenced to some degree, so the meridian system and our psychology are closely linked. EFT is designed to directly interact with the energy system, rebalancing and stabilizing the disruption that occurs

69

when a distressing emotion is experienced, thus enabling our energies to flow freely again.

An EFT session involves gently tapping with the fingertips on specific meridian points on the body, in a set sequence. This simple yet powerful technique rebalances the energies of the body, releasing unwanted emotions and allowing an inner sense of calm to return. Perhaps one of the most amazing effects of EFT is the speed with which emotional distress can be resolved, sometimes in little more than minutes, creating freedom from emotional problems or issues that might have troubled you for years. There are several excellent books that describe this technique in detail – notably *Emotional Healing in Minutes* by Valerie and Paul Lynch, and *The Healing Power of EFT and Energy Psychology* by David Feinstein, Donna Eden and Gary Craig. I highly recommend them if you are interested in learning more. However, as this is such a simple technique I have included the instructions below. Although it looks quite lengthy, that's just because describing it in writing requires rather more explanation – actually, it only takes a few minutes.

The technique is divided into ten steps, split into four stages, and it is important to remember to follow them in progression in order to achieve the desired results. (You may find it useful to write the various stages and your results in a notebook.)

The four stages are:

1. The Set-up
2. The Sequence
3. The Gamut
4. The Second Sequence

1. The Set-up

Step 1, Identify the Problem

Identify the emotion you want to work on, and spend a few moments tuning in to the thoughts and feelings it causes.

Step 2, Formulate a Statement

To establish the intention of what needs to be cleared, you need to create a statement that encompasses these feelings, being as specific, honest and realistic as possible about how you are feeling. The more exact you can be, the deeper the healing can be, because the statement you use needs to have impact and register a disruption within your energy system. So, for example, it is better to be truthful and say something like, 'I am afraid of being hurt if I get involved in a relationship', rather than 'I want to have a loving relationship', because the former statement will generate more emotion.

Therefore to formulate the perfect statement, you need to be as specific as possible, and use the present tense and describe how you feel right now, rather than what you are hoping to achieve. For instance, if you wanted to work on the emotion of anger, you could just say 'I feel angry', but it would be better to be more precise and state why you feel angry, for example, 'I feel angry that my partner won't listen to me' or 'I feel angry that Tom (or Jenny) let me down'.

Next, place the words 'Even though I ...' in front of your chosen statement, followed by '... I deeply and completely accept myself.' For example: 'Even though I feel angry that my partner wouldn't listen to me, I deeply and completely accept myself', 'Even though I am frightened of flying, I deeply and completely accept myself' or 'Even though I am afraid to speak up and say how I feel, I deeply and completely accept myself'.

This type of affirmation promotes acceptance of the problem, and of yourself, and it overrides any part of you that does not want to change, or that has a hidden agenda to keep you the way you are. The statement really needs to be said aloud for the best results, and as emphatically as possible, putting some emotion into it, but if you need to work on something when you're with other people, you can say it silently to yourself.

Step 3, Score Chart

Now you need to get what is called the SUDS level – the Subjective Unit of Distress – by giving your emotion a score from one to ten, relating to its intensity and to how disturbing the memory is, ten being the highest intensity of feeling and zero being the lowest, which means the problem has gone. The score helps you to check and record your progress after the first round, and after any succeeding rounds. As an example, a dreadful trauma or a deeply ingrained fear might be described as an intense 'ten out of ten' reaction, whereas a mild irritation or a slight anxiety might only score a three.

Write down the emotion you want to deal with:

_____

Then put a tick or a cross against the number you feel is appropriate, in the Initial Intensity column:

Initial Intensity	After 1st Round	After 2nd Round	After 3rd Round
10	10	10	10
9	9	9	9
8	8	8	8
7	7	7	7
6	6	6	6
5	5	5	5
4	4	4	4
3	3	3	3
2	2	2	2
1	1	1	1
0	0	0	0

You may not need to go through three rounds, but it's still a good idea to give yourself that number of columns, just in case.

Step 4, Affirmation Link-up

To make the affirmation more effective and give it more energy, *one* of the following two procedures needs to be performed, so experiment and see which you prefer:

A. LOCATING THE TENDER POINTS

Just below your collarbone are the K27 points (see diagram, page 75). You'll probably feel a slight indentation there, and they may feel tender or sore (lymphatic congestion often occurs at these points). Gently rub the two sore spots in a circular motion while repeating your affirmation aloud three times.

B. THE KARATE CHOP POINT

The karate chop points are located on the side of each hand, roughly an inch below the little finger (see diagram, page 76). Gently tap either point with your fingertips for as long as it takes to repeat your affirmation aloud three times.

2. The Sequence

This is the part of the EFT process where the energetic disruption from the body is cleared by tapping all the major meridian points.

Step 5, Reminder Phrase

You need a short reminder phrase to keep your attention focused on the problem, which is said aloud each time you tap every one of the meridian points. This is a shortened version of your affirmation, so it might be 'This nervous feeling', or 'This anger' or 'This hurt'.

Step 6, Tapping Points

Using two fingers, gently but firmly tap each of the meridian points approximately seven times each, from 1 through to 12 in sequence, while repeating your reminder phrase. You can tap with either hand, on either side of the body – or even switch halfway through if you want.

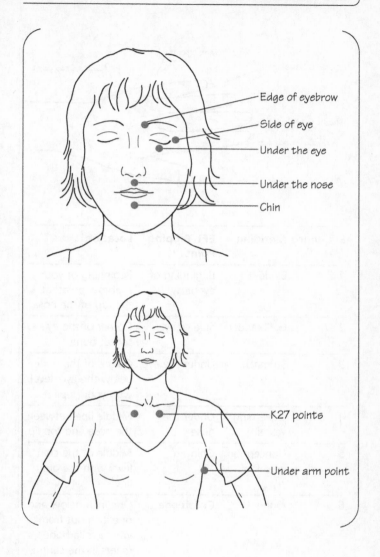

Edge of eyebrow

Side of eye

Under the eye

Under the nose

Chin

K27 points

Under arm point

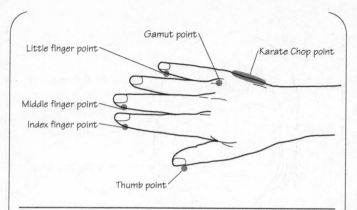

Sequence	Meridian	EFT Tapping Point	Location
1	Bladder	Beginning of eyebrow	Beginning of your eyebrow point, at the top of the nose
2	Gallbladder	Side of eye	Corner of the eye socket bone
3	Stomach	Under the eye	Centre of the bone below the eye, level with your pupil
4	Governing vessel	Under the nose	Middle line between the nose and top lip
5	Conception vessel	Chin	Middle of the chin, level with the gum line
6	Kidney	Collarbone	One inch below and one inch out from where collarbone meets in the centre, just below the neck

7	Spleen	Under arm	On the torso, under the arm, level with nipple (men) or seam of bra (women)
8	Lung	Thumb	Outside edge of thumb, level with base of thumbnail
9	Large intestine	Index finger	Side edge of index finger (nearest to thumb) level with base of fingernail
10	Circulation/ sex	Middle finger	Side of middle finger (nearest to thumb) level with base of fingernail
11	Heart	Little finger	Side of little finger (nearest to thumb), level with base of fingernail
12	Small intestine	Side of hand	Karate chop point, on side of hand, one inch below little finger

When you have completed this sequence, close your eyes and take a deep breath in and out.

13	Triple warmer	Back of hand (Gamut)	On the back of the hand, one centimetre below the knuckles between the ring and little fingers
14	Liver	Under breast	The liver point is not used in EFT

3. The Gamut

Step 7, The Gamut

The Gamut point is on the back of the hand, one centimetre below the knuckles between the ring finger and little fingers. Tap this point at the same time as performing the eye movements below:

EYE MOVEMENTS

1. Close your eyes.
2. Open your eyes.
3. While holding your head still, look hard down right.
4. While holding your head still, look hard down left.
5. While holding your head still, look hard down right again.
6. While holding your head still, look hard down left again.
7. Keeping your head still, roll your eyes in an anti-clockwise direction.
8. Keeping your head still, roll your eyes in a clock-wise direction.

Take a deep breath in and out, and allow a few moments for your energy to reconfigure.

(These eye movements may seem a strange thing to do, but research suggests that our thoughts, memories, feelings, sensations, sounds and visual images all have their individual storage areas in the brain, and these different mental functions can be accessed by means of certain eye positions.)

4. The Second Sequence

Step 8, Second Sequence

When you have completed the Gamut procedure, the tapping sequence is repeated a second time, starting from the eyebrow point, through to the karate chop point, repeating the reminder phrase as before.

Step 9, Reassessment

The first round of EFT is now complete, so it is time to check how you are feeling about your original problem by again giving it a score out of ten (in the first round column), to see if there is any difference. Sometimes there will be a huge change, say from ten down to three or two or even zero, but at other times less difference is noted, say from a starting point of eight, down to six or five.

Step 10, Round Adjustments

Depending on the depth of the problem, the emotional intensity level may drop a few points, so if your original feelings are slightly improved but still present, you will need to repeat the EFT round until the feelings resolve, which may take one or two or more further rounds. When performing repeat round adjustments, you need to make slight changes to your initial statement, which tells the unconscious mind that you now wish to clear the remaining feelings that are connected to the problem, rather than the original feelings you had. You can do this by adding the word 'still'. For example: 'Even though I still feel anger, I deeply and completely accept myself', 'Even though I still feel afraid, I deeply and completely accept myself' or 'Even though I still feel hurt, I deeply and completely accept myself'.

Then repeat the whole process from Step 1 through to Step 9, only this time when tapping using a reminder phrase that includes the word 'remaining', such as: 'This remaining anger', 'This remaining fear' or 'This remaining guilt'.

At this stage you may also find that a completely new aspect or feeling about the same problem surfaces, which is quite common. If this does happen, you may need to formulate a new statement that takes account of the new feeling, and start a whole new EFT round.

Effects During EFT

As you work through the tapping positions you may get a range of physical indications that there is an energy shift going on, such as a need to sigh or yawn or burp (embarrassing but beneficial!), or a feeling of sleepiness or light-headedness. Alternatively, you may experience some emotional indications, such as a feeling of elation or calmness, or sometimes momentary bewilderment or confusion (this soon passes).

A typical EFT session might go like this:

Intensity Score	Reaction	EFT Rounds
10	Terror	1st round
8	Fear	2nd round
6	Apprehension/nervousness	
4	Uncertainty	3rd round
2	Aversion/dislike	
0	Indifference	

If relief doesn't happen immediately after a few rounds of EFT, the changes may still take place over the following few hours or days, which can be because the body needs extra time to incorporate the adjustments that have been made before any of the benefits become apparent. According to Valerie and Paul Lynch, people often achieve insight into their limitations, situations or emotions, and discover where they originated. This is probably because once the emotional charge is reduced, it is possible to see your circumstances more clearly, and with a more balanced outlook, so you might suddenly realize why you feel a certain way, or recognize the original cause of your problem.

Working with EFT

What Gary Craig believed was that the cause of all negative emotions was a disruption in the body's energy system, so using EFT takes away the pain of negative emotions, but leaves insights and memories. Although a specific problem may really need only one or two meridians activating, his reasoning was that if you tap on all the relevant points, then you're bound to do the ones you need. Essentially, this works because your body probably received programming, e.g. fear of spiders or fear of rejection, when you were small or at another time when you were under severe stress or going through trauma, but it is possible for you to reprogramme it. Basically the process is to tap out the negative, and then (if necessary) tap in the positive.

Complete beginners can usually achieve 50 per cent success, and experienced practitioners between 80 and 98 per cent success, because the wording is important, and that's what needs practice. If you follow the process above, you can do it on yourself, but you might also consider going to an EFT practitioner, or taking a course in EFT. There are some contact addresses given in Useful Addresses, page 251.

Having examined emotions in general, in the next chapter we look in more detail at anger and how to cope with it.

chapter six

DEALING WITH ANGER

At the beginning of the last chapter, I referred to Dr Usui's first Principle, 'just for today, do not anger', and as I mentioned, initially this may seem an almost impossible request. What I hope to show you in this chapter is that it is possible to handle your anger in different ways, and even to reduce the number of times you feel angry, until you reach a stage where you are calm and centred enough not to feel anger in any but the most extreme circumstances.

WHAT IS ANGER?

Anger is 'an emotional state that varies in intensity from mild irritation to intense fury and rage', according to Charles Spielberger, PhD, a psychologist who specializes in the study of anger. An angry response may sometimes feel like the only option, but anger can be a very destructive emotion, and often it hurts us almost as much as it hurts those against whom we direct it, as they are often the people we care about the most. Anger is usually triggered when someone or something fails to meet our expectations, and sometimes – even more importantly –

when we don't come up to our own expectations. However, like any other emotion, anger is actually a conscious choice, a habitual response you have developed, as mentioned in Chapter 5. Expressing anger towards someone rarely achieves anything other than to make you both feel bad, but you *can* break the cycle and choose a different response instead. You can find healthier and safer ways of expressing the frustration that usually lies behind the anger by turning the emotion into creativity, going for a brisk walk or doing that very old-fashioned thing, counting to ten before you speak! Sometimes a short pause is all it takes to defuse a situation and allow you to talk calmly, in an assertive and adult way, rather than sliding into belligerence and aggressiveness.

The next time you feel angry, pause for a moment and ask yourself 'why?' What is going on? Is this a replay of something that has happened over and over again? Are you angry about the thing you think you're angry about – such as a partner's insulting comment in front of your friends – or is there something deeper going on, like a general dissatisfaction with your relationship? It's only by asking yourself these sorts of questions that you will begin to unravel the issues which are triggering the emotion of anger and begin the healing process.

A Reiki Technique for Revealing Causes

This technique can generate insight and intuition about the causes of problems, and also helps to calm you down and promote healing of the situation.

1. Decide what situation you want to work on that is generating feelings of anger in you. Continue to think about it throughout the treatment, and let yourself be open to receiving intuition or insight into the causes.

2. Sit or lie down and place one hand at the back of your neck and one on the front of your throat, and let Reiki flow for your greatest and highest good for about five minutes, or longer if you feel this is necessary.

3. Place one (or both) hands on your crown, and let Reiki flow for five minutes or more.

4. Place one hand on your stomach (solar plexus) and the other over your intestines (navel area), and hold your hands there for five minutes or more.

5. Remove your hands, gassho (i.e. place your hands in the prayer position in front of the centre of your chest, see page 15), give thanks for the Reiki and end with a bow of respect.

6. Spend a few minutes sitting quietly, contemplating any insight or intuition you discovered, and thinking about how this might help you to resolve the situation.

THE PHYSIOLOGY OF ANGER

Like other emotions, anger is accompanied by physiological and biological changes similar to those our prehistoric ancestors experienced as a reaction to danger – what is known as the 'fight-or-flight response'. When you get angry, your body can experience any of the following reactions, depending on the level of emotion you're feeling:

- Increase in heart rate and blood pressure.
- Constriction of blood vessels in some areas of the body.
- Increase in blood sugar levels.
- Redirection of blood flow away from extremities towards major organs.
- Faster and deeper breathing.
- Digestion stops or slows down.
- Increased sweating.

These transformations are the result of neurohormonal changes, especially the production in the adrenal glands of adrenaline and noradrenaline, which circulate in the bloodstream and target various organs, such as the heart to increase its rate of beating. Another neurohormonal system also located in the adrenal glands stimulates increased secretion of corticosteroids, especially cortisol, which help to prepare the body for action by increasing the release of glucose and other fuels from stores within the body. This is one of the reasons why an angry response can sometimes escalate into physical action – fighting or brawling – because (literally) your 'blood is up' and you are ready for anything.

The instinctive, natural way to express anger is thus to respond aggressively. Anger is a natural, adaptive response to threats, which inspires powerful, often aggressive, feelings and behaviours that allow us to fight and defend ourselves when we are attacked. A certain amount of anger, therefore, is necessary to our survival.

Of course, in our ancestors these reactions were always meant to be a short-term answer to an emergency, like running away from a sabre-tooth tiger or fighting off an enemy tribe, but in Western society we are rarely in extreme physical danger, so our 'stressors' or 'anger triggers' are more likely to be psychological in origin. Again, these might be of short duration, but the kind of stress that many people can identify with in modern society tends to be ongoing, chronic and long term, and this often results in decreased tolerance and increased frustration, and a consequent 'short fuse' for our tempers.

If your body is constantly on the alert because of chronic stress – and frequent episodes of anger actually add to the stress load – this ceases to be an adaptive condition and can lead to health problems. The state of heightened physical arousal that anger can induce puts considerable strain on our bodies, and chronic sustained anger can cause or exacerbate digestive disorders such as ulcers and gastritis, create hypertension, raise cholesterol levels, aggravate heart disease, exacerbate bowel conditions and affect the immune system, among other things. Anger therefore isn't a very healthy emotion to have, at least if it is experienced frequently.

EXPERIENCING ANGER

Some of the most common causes of anger include hurt or indignation, frustration or irritation, harassment or persecution, disappointment or regret, and perceived threats. However, the source of all of these feelings is based on unfulfilled expectations, and if you can let go of

87

your expectations, you will be able to let go of your anger. Before you can get to that stage, you might need some help just handling the feelings you are already experiencing.

There are basically two ways of experiencing anger:

1. You can feel angry with yourself in a variety of ways. Perhaps you haven't done as well as you had hoped in a job interview or examination, or you feel you've let someone down, or you've let yourself down by being late again for an important meeting, or you've lost something, and so on.

2. You can have the other kind of anger which is directed at someone else or some object – so you might be angry with your partner as a result of an argument, or as a reaction to something they've done, or you could be angry with a sales person for not being helpful enough, with a work colleague because they've 'messed up' in some way or even with the dishwasher because it has broken down.

Some people describe these two ways as:

1. Internal anger that is directed at yourself for something that you have done, or have not done.

2. External anger that is the result of an interaction with another person.

However, these aren't accurate descriptions – both types of anger are actually internally generated, and no one has ever *made* you angry. It has all been your own work! Anger is just one of a whole range of responses you could have to a given set of circumstances, which means it is a choice you have made, even if it doesn't feel like it. That's quite empowering, because if you can choose anger as a response, it also means you can choose some other response instead. There's a phrase I was introduced to many years ago by a colleague, and I've never forgotten it: 'If you always do what you've always done, you will always get what you've always got.'

In other words, if your habitual response to a given set of circumstances is always the same – such as always reacting angrily when your partner does something you don't like – you will always get the same sort of response from them, which will probably be defensive, or perhaps mirror your own anger because they feel threatened by it. See what I mean? If you can change *your* reaction by perhaps being more understanding of the other person's position because you realize their perception of it is different to yours, or feeling less threatened by someone's actions by developing more self-confidence and greater self-esteem, or simply by listening to their explanation rather than instantly 'sounding off', then you'll get a whole new set of reactions from the people around you.

EXPRESSING ANGER

When we experience anger we can't always physically or verbally lash out at every person or object that irritates or annoys us – laws, social norms and common sense place limits on how far our anger can take us. People use a variety of both conscious and unconscious processes to deal with their angry feelings, the three main approaches being:

◆ Expressing
◆ Suppressing
◆ Calming

Expressing your angry feelings in an assertive − not aggressive − manner is the healthiest way. To do this, you have to learn how to make clear what your needs are, and how to get them met, without hurting others. Being assertive doesn't mean being pushy or demanding; it means being respectful of yourself and others.

I am not advocating that you should always vent your feelings directly on the person who has triggered angry emotions in you. That can be unwise and even unhealthy − especially if their reaction is likely to be to punch you on the nose! Anger can be suppressed at the moment it is experienced, then converted or redirected. You can do this by holding in your anger, ceasing to think about it and focusing on something positive. The aim is to inhibit or suppress your anger, at least for a while, and convert it into more constructive behaviour. The problem with this type of response is that if it isn't allowed outward expression at some point, your anger can turn inwards, which can potentially cause high blood pressure, or even depression. It can also lead to passive-aggressive behaviour, such as getting back at people indirectly, without telling them why, rather than confronting them head-on. People who are constantly putting others down, criticizing everything and making cynical comments almost certainly haven't learned how to constructively express their anger.

However, it is possible to cool down, which means not only controlling your outward behaviour, but also controlling your internal responses and taking steps to lower your heart rate, calm yourself down and let the feelings subside.

COPING WITH ANGRY FEELINGS

The goal of anger management is to allow you to deal with your anger at a comfortable pace, in a way that helps to resolve the situation and doesn't create worse problems. I suggested earlier that it would be a good idea to ask yourself why you're feeling angry, but of course at the moment that emotion is aroused, you might think you are much less able to be objective, and certainly less able to be reflective. However, the human thought process is incredibly fast, so it is possible to think through the following stages in a matter of seconds. Before you speak or do anything else:

- Recognize and admit your feelings of anger.
- Identify the target and cause of your anger.
- Consider as many options as possible for responding to the situation, together with their possible results.
- Choose the best option – and follow it through.

Let's look at these stages one at a time. Firstly, recognizing and admitting to yourself that you feel angry is important because it means you are actually considering how you feel, rather than just reacting as if on 'auto-pilot'. You are thinking through what is happening, not just letting rip with your first instinctive (habitual) response. Maybe using an example would be helpful here.

Your boss has just dumped a huge load of work on your desk, saying it all has to be done today, but there's only half an hour left of your normal working day, so you know you're being asked to work late again, and it's the third time this week. You feel angry.

Now let's identify the target and cause of your anger.

The immediate target is obviously your boss (although it might be that they have only just had the work dumped on them by their boss!), but the causes might be a lot harder to identify. You might feel resentful because you had other plans, or hurt because you feel you're being taken advantage of, or disgusted because you know your boss is disorganized and could have given you the work earlier, or furious because you don't think you're being paid enough to take this level of responsibility. Identifying what underlies your anger is a really useful step, because it will help you to realize what to do about it.

Then you need to consider what your options are in terms of responding to the situation, and theorize about what results they might have.

- You could react angrily, shout at your boss, refuse to do the work and storm out, throwing the words 'I quit' behind you, if they haven't already said 'You're fired'. Not the most productive reaction, as you've just lost your job!

- You could swallow your anger, not say anything to your boss about your plans, and work as fast as you can, not really caring too much if you make mistakes, and leave an hour late, all the time feeling resentful, angry, put upon and generally wishing your boss would fall down a big hole. Again, not very productive, because you haven't got rid of the angry feelings: you've just pushed them down, so they're still simmering away, waiting to erupt – which they'll probably do as soon as you get home, which isn't going to be nice for your partner/ family/dog/cat! Also, you've ended up doing something you don't want to do, which is unsatisfactory and will just add to the burden the next time you're called upon to work late.

- You could do whatever you can in your last half-hour, then just pick up your coat and leave, without saying anything to the boss. However, then you have to face up to the boss the next morning, so you'll probably worry about that all night.

- You could do whatever you can in the time, or stay and finish the work, but recognize that this is an ongoing situation and plan to complain to someone about the amount of work you are expected to do. Perhaps your company has a Human Resources section or union you can turn to, or maybe you could get other members of staff on your side, as it's unlikely you're the only one who is having to do more work than is possible in a day. Any of those possibilities could have repercussions, of course, and you wouldn't be making yourself popular with your boss, but sometimes someone needs to stand up for what they believe is right, and that someone may have to be you.

◆ You could say quietly but firmly that you have to leave on time today as you have plans for the evening, so you will get done as much as you can in the next half-hour. You might also suggest that your boss could prioritize the most urgent work in the pile, and you'll start immediately on that, and maybe some of the work could be passed over to other staff members if there are any. Being assertive, rather than aggressive, is often the best response, and surprisingly often engenders much more respect from employers than submissive behaviour. Of course, it is a risk – some employers won't react favourably, but standing up for yourself will usually make you feel better about yourself than meekly giving in. There is really no excuse for bosses who take advantage of their employees' good nature – it's exploitative.

◆ And of course, you could send Reiki to the situation. See the simple method below.

Those are just a few ideas for dealing with one situation, but your situation may be completely different, and need alternative ways of coping, but hopefully you'll find something helpful in the process I've illustrated.

SENDING REIKI TO A SITUATION

The easiest way to do this is to write down your circumstances on a piece of paper, such as: 'let Reiki flow to the situation of my boss giving me extra work too late in the day', and hold the paper between your hands, allowing Reiki to flow into it for at least 5–10 minutes, or until you begin to notice a change in the way you feel about it. (If you have Reiki Second Degree, you can draw the Distant symbol in the air over the paper to connect to the situation, then draw the Harmony symbol to bring peace and harmony to the situation and finally draw the Power symbol to bring the Reiki in.) Sometimes using Reiki in this way actually produces insight into the best way to deal with the situation, but because the Reiki will also flow to your boss's Higher Self, it can impact on the way they behave, too. Try it – it can be amazingly powerful!

SAFER WAYS OF EXPRESSING ANGER

Basically you have choices to make. You can express your anger directly and verbally – which is sometimes risky, but if you are polite, don't shout and own the anger, that is you don't blame the other person, and don't just 'blow up', it can sometimes work well. By 'owning' the anger I mean saying 'I am feeling angry about what you've just said/done', rather than saying 'You've really made me angry now' – because the other person hasn't made you angry, you've just chosen to react that way. You can then go on to discuss in a calmer and more adult way what it is about what they've said or done that you don't like, so there's then a chance to resolve the state of affairs.

Sometimes using humour will help to defuse a situation, or you might want to let whatever it is pass this time, giving yourself time to think it through properly so you know how to face up to it next time it happens. Often it's a good idea to look at the situation in a different way. Try putting yourself in the other person's place to see if you can understand why they are doing or saying something; no one's perspective on the world is the same as anyone else's, so maybe there are things going on in that person's life that you don't know about, and that are making them behave the way they are.

Perhaps you need to talk over your feelings with someone you trust – a friend or counsellor – to get a different perspective on the issue, because if bad situations go on for a long time it's easy to get things out of proportion, but not easy to see that's what we've done, so a neutral third party can really help us to 'see the wood from the trees'.

Sometimes just letting out a scream of frustration (obviously somewhere private!) or slamming a door can help to release the tension. If you've had a bad day at work and travelled in your own car, use the drive home as an opportunity to say out loud all those things you wish you'd been able to say, as if the source of the aggravation was with you, so that by the time you get home you've 'got it off your chest' and can get on with the rest of your day with a smile. If you're travelling home on public transport where talking aloud wouldn't be an option, you could close your eyes and imagine yourself saying what you wanted to say, and imagine the situation being resolved happily. Or maybe you need to let out the day's annoyances by doing something physical, like jogging, cycling or swimming. You can of course also choose to let go of the issue, and decide that it isn't worth getting angry about – another version of this Principle is 'just for today, I will let go of anger!'

There are other things you can do to help cope with anger, such as deep breathing (see page 41), giving yourself Reiki for a few minutes to help to calm you (see page 68), going somewhere private and carrying out a Reiki Shower, a technique for imagining Reiki flowing over your whole body to flush away negativity and unwanted emotions (see below), or meditating quietly until you receive some insight on the problem. They might not be the first things you think of when anger strikes, but as you get better at coping with it, you'll find it easier to be more accepting of other people's attitudes and behaviour, and it will then be easier to take a calmer and more centred approach.

THE REIKI SHOWER

This is a technique from the Japanese tradition that is suitable for anyone with any level of Reiki. It consists of activating and cleansing your whole energy body (within your physical body and outside it throughout your aura) by absorbing Reiki energy like a shower. You can use this technique almost anywhere for cleansing and calming yourself, and it also helps to centre you, raising your consciousness and bringing you into a pleasantly meditative state. It can be carried out either standing or sitting in a chair.

1. Stand or sit, and make yourself comfortable, place your hands in the gassho (prayer) position, with your palms together, fingers pointing upwards, and your hands held close to your body at the level of the heart chakra. Stay like this for a few moments, letting your breathing become slower and deeper, and intend to carry out a Reiki Shower.

2. Then separate your hands and lift them above your head, as high as possible, keeping them about 30 to 40 cm (12–15 in) apart. Wait for a few moments until you begin to feel the Reiki building up between your hands, then turn your palms downwards so that they are facing the top of your head.

3. Visualize Reiki flowing out of your hands, and *intend* that you are receiving a shower of Reiki energy, which flows over and through your whole physical and energy body, cleansing you and removing any negative energy or emotions.

4. When you sense the vibration of the Reiki energy flowing over and through you, move your hands, palms still facing towards you, and begin to draw them slowly down over your face and body, keeping your hands about 30–40 cm (12–15 in) away from your body. *Intend* that Reiki is flowing from your hands, and continuing to cleanse and revitalize you

as you draw your hands all the way down your body, and then down your legs to your feet, eventually turning your palms to face the floor and either touching the floor, or gently throwing the energy off your hands so that any negative energy flows out and into the earth below, for transformation.

6. Repeat this exercise a few times – I find three times to be ideal – and you should feel cleansed, calm and relaxed.

7. Place your hands together again in the gassho position, and spend a few moments experiencing gratitude for the Reiki, and then finish. You may find it helpful to clap your hands once or twice, to help you to return to a more wakeful state if you feel a bit 'spaced'.

OTHER HELPFUL TECHNIQUES

If you have access to the Internet you'll find lots of information on anger management, and there are some good ideas out there. Some of them are old standards, like deep breathing and meditation, but others are newer techniques that are gaining popularity, like forms of acupressure such as EFT (see Chapter 5). There are many books around nowadays on positive psychology and achieving happiness – there are beneficial effects on brain chemistry of being positive, smiling and laughing, so you might choose to read up on that. I would recommend *The Endorphin Effect* by William Bloom, or any of the books by Robert Holden.

Talking about your feelings to someone you know and trust, and who will take you seriously but be supportive, is often a good choice, but sometimes talking directly to the person who triggers your anger is a necessary part of healing the situation between you, because if you never clear the air the situation usually just gets worse. Many people fear hurting someone else's feelings if they share their angry feelings with them, but holding on to anger often makes you behave differently, so the other person ends up feeling hurt anyway, and that can damage the relationship. You just need to be careful how you say things – it's important not to be accusatory or judgemental, and to give the other person a chance to have their say, without you reacting angrily to their thoughts or beliefs.

Each of us has the right to be ourselves, and sometimes huge rows can be the result of very small differences of opinion that could be sorted out quite easily if we could just feel safe with each other. Agreeing to spend time talking things over is the first step towards solving the problem, although sometimes it helps to have a 'neutral' person around as a potential arbiter, such as a relationship counsellor.

Another possibility is to write down your feelings, which is a good way of getting them 'out there', rather than keeping them stuck inside. I would, however, advise that it is not a good idea to let the person you're writing about see what you've written. By all means write them a letter and put in it all the stuff you'd like to say to them – but don't post it. Instead, hold a little ceremony where you symbolically burn the letter (in a safe place, like in a metal saucepan so you can put the lid on afterwards to make sure the flames go out properly) and let the smoke take your anger with it, to be healed and transformed, so you know you have truly let go of the issue.

INDIVIDUAL PERCEPTION

The problem we all have is that we generally only see things from our own perspective, and often assume that the way we see things is the way others see things. This is often at the root cause of problems with interactions with other people, which in turn can lead to the development of negative emotions like anger. Given the same trigger, under the same conditions, some people will laugh off frustration, others will express mild irritation and others still will get into a rage, stamping their feet and shouting. Each person will have perceived the situation differently, and will have reacted in a different way according to how they have individually learned to manage and demonstrate their feelings. There is a Neuro Linguistic Programming (NLP) technique called Perceptual Positions which can help you to consider other viewpoints on an issue or situation.

Neuro Linguistic Programming (NLP)

I trained to became an NLP Practitioner in the 1990s, and have found many of the techniques to be really helpful as an addition to my Reiki practice, so this is something I'd like to introduce to you. NLP was developed in the mid-seventies by a linguist, John Grinder, and a mathematician, Richard Bandler, who had strong interests in successful people, psychology, language and computer programming. They developed a range of communication and persuasion techniques, including self-hypnosis, to help people to motivate and change themselves, and create greater self-esteem, by reprogramming their brains. At another level, NLP is about self-discovery, exploring identity and relating to the 'spiritual' part of human experience that reaches beyond us as individuals to our family, community and global systems.

PERCEPTUAL POSITIONS TECHNIQUE

Most NLP techniques are deceptively simple – that is, they create change quickly and easily by reprogramming the way you think. In this technique you are asked to look at a particular situation, such as one that could potentially become an angry exchange between you and a colleague or family member, from three perspectives – Self, Other and Observer – using your imagination to gather information and explore your feelings. This may sound a bit strange, but I can assure you it really works.

Place three pieces of paper on the floor, or just imagine three distinct spaces, as below:

SELF   OTHER

OBSERVER

1. Decide what situation you are going to consider – something that might trigger anger in you – including who the interaction is with, and what subject or situation the two of you might be discussing.

2. First, stand on the SELF space, and think about the situation and get as much information as possible – what do you see, what do you hear, what do you feel?

3. Then move to the OTHER space, and imagine that you are the other person. Now what do you see, what do you hear, what do you feel?

4. Then move to the OBSERVER space, and consider the interaction between SELF and OTHER. As an impartial and benevolent observer, you make no judgements, but simply gather information about the relationship between Self and Other. What do you see, what do you hear, what do you believe is going on?

5. Finally, move back to the SELF space, and allow the insights from the other two perspectives to be integrated into your own perceptions. How have they altered how you see things? How have they altered how you hear things? How have they altered how you feel?

6. Step into a neutral space (i.e. not in one of the three positions), and spend some time assimilating what has happened, perhaps by writing it down, or by sitting quietly and thinking about it. Become aware of new possibilities of behaviour and language that may enable you to achieve your desired outcome and enhance the relationship between you.

STRATEGIES TO KEEP ANGER AT BAY

Learn to be More Tolerant, Compassionate and Accepting

When we get angry, it is usually because we are intolerant of other people's views, beliefs or behaviour, and therefore cannot accept something that someone has said or done – or perhaps their age or gender or sexual orientation, or anything else that is in some way different. Developing tolerance could help us, potentially, to live without anger.

The point is, people who demonstrate what we might call intolerant behaviour generally don't think, feel or believe that they are being intolerant. They see nothing wrong in what they are doing or saying, because it accurately reflects their own concepts and life experience. It is all they know. Every person's life involves developing a value system by which they live. We form our value systems based on our life experience, and that naturally starts with what we see and hear as children, and goes on developing as we become teenagers and then adults. The main problem is that most of us don't realize that other people don't necessarily think or feel the same way we do. However, if we could respect the rights of individuals to be who they are, and develop a strong and positive acceptance of other people's differences, and an appreciation of why those differences exist, we could become more tolerant.

◆ If we could generate a climate of understanding, perhaps people wouldn't feel they had to stick so rigidly to their own ideas, but would recognize that other people's ideas had value too, so some sensible compromises could be reached.

◆ If we could generate a climate of compassion, perhaps we would recognize that everyone becomes the person they are because of the sum of their experiences so far, so maybe then we wouldn't judge others so harshly.

◆ If we could generate a climate of acceptance, perhaps we wouldn't need to feel challenged by people's differences, but instead could all learn to accept that each person is unique, with their own unique way of thinking, feeling and seeing the world, so we wouldn't always expect them to think and behave like us, but instead could accept the strength in variety and diversity.

Learn to be More Forgiving

Forgiveness is the mental and/or spiritual process of ceasing to feel resentment, indignation or anger against another person for a perceived offence, difference or mistake, or ceasing to demand punishment or restitution. In order to forgive someone, you first have to judge that what they have said or done is wrong. Of course, I can almost hear the reactions from some readers – that there are awful things that some people do, which must be wrong. However, we *all* do what we believe is right, at least most of the time, and under certain circumstances we could *all* do things that we currently wouldn't contemplate. For example, however 'civilized' you might think you are, if you are a parent, you would probably be prepared to kill to protect your children if they were under serious threat – it's a basic instinct. If your children were starving and there was no other way, you would probably be prepared to steal food, or money to buy food. You would justify to yourself that those actions were not wrong, under those circumstances. 'There but for the grace of God go I' is a phrase that comes to mind.

Sometimes we do need to 'forgive and forget' to help us to move on. *Beliefs divide us. Emotions can unite us.* While the ideal might be to view everyone as just living their lives the best way they can, and seeing them as 'spirit having a human experience' and just learning whatever they need to learn in this life, we are still human. Sometimes it's tough to try to understand someone else's motivation if they do or say something that hurts us, or hurts those we love. But we can try it just for today. You might find the following visualization helpful.

FORGIVENESS VISUALIZATION

Try this by thinking of one person to start with, although when you've practised it for a while you could visualize a small group of people, such as some members of your family or several work colleagues.

- Settle yourself comfortably and relax by breathing deeply and evenly, and when you are ready, imagine yourself on one side of a fast-flowing river.
- Take some time to make the image as real as you can – it can be a river you know, or one you just imagine – but try to see, feel and smell the whole

---

scene, the grass or sand or pebbles on the riverbank, the blue sky and warm sun, the smell of wild
flowers, the sound of the running water and birdsong.

◆ When you have the picture firmly in mind, look
across to the other side of the river, and see or sense
a person standing there. This is a person with
whom you have felt angry, and whom you have
decided to connect with in this visualization.

◆ Let the picture fill out so that you see what they
are wearing, and maybe see the expression on their
face.

◆ Now ask Reiki and your Higher Self to help you
to develop understanding and forgiveness of this
person, and of yourself, and see or sense a bridge
beginning to form between you, over the river.

◆ It may be very wispy to begin with, but gradually
a good, strong bridge is created. It may appear to
be made of brick or stone, wood or metal, or it
may even consist of stepping stones, but now there
is a connection between the two sides of the river.

◆ If it still doesn't look solid, ask Reiki and your
Higher Self to help again by giving you confidence
and allowing you to trust the process. (If you have
Reiki Second Degree, you can imagine the Distant
symbol stretching out in front of you to create the
bridge.)

◆ Next, step onto the bridge, and begin to walk
across it, but pause in the middle. Hopefully the
person on the other side has also started to walk

across it towards you, but if not, just wait a little longer.

- Then imagine Reiki flowing out of your hands and filling your aura, and spreading out in front of you across the bridge to encompass and enfold the other person in Reiki, and ask Reiki to heal the differences between you, to create harmony and calm. (You can imagine the Harmony symbol for this, too.)

- When you can meet in the middle of the bridge, which is a neutral space for you both, allow the other person to say whatever they need to say, without judging it. You are talking soul to soul, so what the other person says is the truth as they know it, even if it is not the same as the truth as you see it.

- When they have finished talking, speak your truth to them, and ask that Reiki flow into the situation to help you to create an atmosphere of forgiveness and trust. This may take a few minutes, but be patient, and eventually you will feel a spread of calmness throughout your body, and you will know that you have forgiven each other at a soul level.

- Imagine yourselves shaking hands, or hugging each other, as appropriate, and smile, thanking them for being present, and thanking Reiki and your Higher Selves for being present and helping in this situation.

- Turn and walk back to your side of the river, step off the bridge and let the bridge slowly dissolve.

- Wave and smile at the person on the other side of the bank, then gradually let your awareness of the present return, as you feel the chair or bed beneath you, and hear the sounds in the room.
- Finally, write down what you have experienced, so that you can reach even greater insight and understanding at a later date.

Learn to Calm Down and Relax

If you feel yourself getting angry, don't let the feeling build up until you have a violent outburst; try to calm down and relax instead. If you find it difficult to relax, there are books and courses that can help, but simple relaxation tools, such as deep breathing and relaxing visualizations, can be an aid to calming angry feelings. Here are some simple steps you can try. If you practise them regularly, you'll be able to use them automatically when you're in a tense situation.

- Breathe deeply, into your diaphragm, hold your breath for as long as is comfortable, then release it quite quickly, and you will find that your whole body relaxes.
- Visualize yourself in a beautiful place, like a woodland glade, or sitting beside a lake, or on a mountain-top with wonderful views around you, and hold that image in your mind until you feel yourself calming down.
- Do some non-strenuous, slow stretching (yoga exercises), which can relax your muscles and make you feel calmer.

Learn to Express Yourself Calmly and Assertively

Try to express angry feelings in an assertive manner, using calm, logical words rather than violence. If you are having, or expecting to have, a heated discussion, slow down – think carefully about what you want to say, be clear about what you are asking and how it can be achieved and listen carefully to the other person, remembering that everyone is entitled to their own opinion. We all have our own communication style, which can be just a habit, or could be something we've copied from the way our parents or other adults spoke when we were children.

Most communication styles can be classified as aggressive, non-assertive or assertive.

Aggressive

Anger often results in aggressive behaviour, but whether this is expressed directly or indirectly it always communicates an impression of superiority and disrespect. By being aggressive we put our wants, needs and rights above those of others, and we attempt to get our way by not allowing others a choice, so it is often seen as bullying.

Examples: 'That was a stupid thing to do.' 'You're always interrupting me.'

Non-assertive

This is passive and indirect, and it communicates a message of inferiority. By being non-assertive we allow the wants, needs and rights of others to be more important than our own.

Examples: 'I'm not very good at this sort of thing.' 'Well, all right, if that's what you want to do.'

Assertive

Being assertive, rather than aggressive, communicates an impression of self-respect and respect for others. By being assertive we view our wants, needs and rights as equal with those of others. We work towards 'win–win' outcomes (i.e. those that are successful for each party). An assertive person wins by influencing, listening and negotiating, so that others choose to cooperate willingly. This behaviour leads to success without retaliation, and encourages honest, open relationships.

Examples: 'I'm sorry I can't go, I have other plans.' 'That idea might not work, so perhaps we could look at some other options together.'

Assertiveness requires us to accept responsibility for our thoughts, feelings and behaviour, and requires us to respect the thoughts, feelings and behaviour of others. You cannot be solely responsible for the feelings of others because you do not 'make them feel'. You are responsible for what you say and do because your words and actions invite others to feel certain emotions, but what they feel is up to them. When an individual accepts these responsibilities and stops blaming others for his or her feelings, they have taken a giant step towards communicating in a sensible, adult way.

To communicate thoughts, feelings and opinions assertively, you need to choose words that are direct, honest, appropriate and respectful.

◆ Use 'I statements' rather than 'you statements', and own your own feelings rather than blaming someone else. Example: 'I felt unhappy when you said that' rather than 'what you said made me feel unhappy'.

- Use factual descriptions instead of judgements or exaggerations. Example: 'this letter needs retyping because some punctuation is missing' rather than 'this work is rubbish'.
- Use clear, direct requests or directives (commands) when you want others to do something, rather than hinting, being indirect or presuming. Example: 'please make three copies of this document' rather than 'I need three copies of this document'.

Learn a New Lifestyle

Some aspects of our lifestyles can lead to more frequent problems with anger, so by making some helpful changes you can reap great benefits:

- Take regular exercise – walking, cycling, swimming – to help to work off tension and stress.
- Take part in yoga or meditation classes to help to release tension in a controlled, healthy way.
- Eat healthily, including plenty of fresh vegetables and fruits in your diet, and cutting out as many additives and preservatives as you can, as these can have detrimental effects on your mood.
- Keep your alcohol consumption within the daily recommended intake of 2–3 units for women and 3–4 units for men. Alcohol lowers your inhibitions, which can trigger violent behaviour.
- Spend as little time as possible in stressful environments or with people who affect you negatively, and schedule some time for relaxation and unwinding.
- Express your feelings in healthy ways, either by talking to a friend or creatively through painting or writing.

SEEKING HELP FOR ANGER OR AGGRESSION

Some people need more help than others to address their anger or aggression problem, but if that includes you, don't feel embarrassed about seeking professional help. People who are angry and aggressive do need to take responsibility for their actions – blaming others isn't helpful – but looking back at your past might help you to understand your current angry behaviour. For example, if your parents or other family members set bad examples and resolved conflicts angrily or aggressively, you might not have learned to deal with anger constructively. It is possible to change your anger patterns, and professional services can help to improve anger management.

You might consider going on a course to learn more about how to be assertive, rather than aggressive, and your local library or further education college might have details of suitable classes.

Counselling or Cognitive Behavioural Therapy (looking at how you think and behave) can help you to look at your thinking and behaviour associated with anger, and you could find a suitable therapist through your doctor. They might also direct you to an anger management programme, which could be a weekend course or regular evening sessions including both one-to-one and group work.

USE THE REIKI PRINCIPLES AS AFFIRMATIONS

If you keep repeating the phrase to yourself 'just for today, do not anger', when you feel yourself becoming irritated, that can help. You can also turn it into a positive affirmation, and keep telling yourself 'today I will be cool, calm and relaxed', and that can be even more beneficial.

To conclude, you will always come across situations that could potentially provoke anger, but the key is to take responsibility for your own reactions and behaviour by addressing angry feelings with new coping mechanisms and responses, using the various Reiki techniques and other methods described in this chapter and Chapter 5, which I hope will, eventually, lead to you 'living without anger'.

In Part 4, we look at the second of Dr Usui's Principles, 'just for today, do not worry', and consider the power of thought, and how it is possible to stop worrying and start living.

part four

LIVING WITHOUT WORRY

Worry wounds the body,
Contemplation heals the mind,
Meditation unites the spirit.
Revd Simon John Barlow

chapter seven

UNDERSTANDING THOUGHTS, AND THE POWER OF WORDS

'Just for today, do not worry' is the second of the Principles passed on to us by Dr Usui, and for many this also may seem a difficult, if not impossible, request. Some people are described as 'born worriers', and the way they react to life is to agonize about almost everything – even to the extent of worrying that they haven't got anything to worry about! What I hope to show you in this and the next chapter is that worrying can be a habit, and like any habit, it is possible to break it, so you can change your thinking patterns to be more positive, which is a happier and healthier alternative. Chapter 8 examines worry in more depth, but worry is just one form of thinking that can disturb our mental state and make it more difficult to 'live the Reiki way', so first we look at the process of thinking, as it controls so much of what we say and do.

THE BRAIN AND THINKING

Thought or thinking is a mental process that allows you to model the world, or, in other words, to bring the world into focus in a way that you can make sense of, which helps you to deal with it effectively. A thought may be an idea, image, sound, smell or touch, or even an emotional feeling that arises from the brain, because it is usually your thoughts that generate your emotions. When you are thinking, your brain is manipulating information, which is what is happening when you form concepts and engage in problem solving, reasoning and making decisions. Other brain functions include arousal, attention, concentration, consciousness, language, learning, memory, motor coordination, perception and planning. There are three parts to your brain:

1. The brain stem, or physical (reptilian) brain, which acts on a subconscious level and controls such things as breathing, heart rate, muscles and sleep, and any instinctive processes, such as reacting to danger.
2. The limbic or emotional brain, which controls emotions and motivation, and also acts as a filter for all the information your brain receives (which is why it is easier to remember things that happened when your emotions were aroused, either positively, when you were happy or successful, or negatively, when you were sad or frightened).
3. The cerebral cortex, or thinking brain, which is divided into two halves: the left hemisphere, which is responsible for logic, analysis, fact, language, mathematics and sequence thinking, and the right

hemisphere, which is responsible for creative thinking, rhyme, rhythm, music, pictures, daydreaming and visualizing.

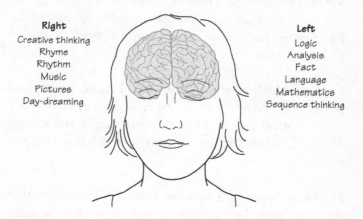

Right
Creative thinking
Rhyme
Rhythm
Music
Pictures
Day-dreaming

Left
Logic
Analysis
Fact
Language
Mathematics
Sequence thinking

There has been a lot of research into the different functions of the two halves of your thinking brain, and people sometimes describe themselves as either 'left brain thinkers' or 'right brain thinkers'. While this can certainly be a useful image to use, in reality it's not correct, because everyone has the ability to use both parts of their brain, although each of us does seem to have one side that is slightly more dominant.

Thinking Styles

Whichever hemisphere of our brain we consider might be dominant, we don't all think in the same way. An important aspect of our personalities and the way we react to the world is our thinking style, and you might like to have a guess at which style of the following nine you feel most at home with, although most of us probably reflect two or three styles, with one being more frequently used.

Verbal/Linguistic Thinkers Tend to think in words, like to use language to express complex ideas, and are sensitive to the sounds and rhythms of words as well as their meanings.

Logical/Mathematical Thinkers Like to understand patterns and relationships between objects or actions, try to understand the world in terms of causes and effects, and are good at thinking critically and solving problems creatively.

Musical/Creative Thinkers Feel a strong connection between music and emotions, tend to think in sounds, may also think in rhythms and melodies, and are sensitive to the sounds and rhythms of words as well as their meanings.

Spatial/Visual Thinkers Tend to think in pictures, think well in three dimensions, have a flair for working with objects, and can develop good mental models of the physical world.

Body/Kinaesthetic Thinkers Tend to think in movements, so they like to use their bodies in skilful and expressive ways, and have an aptitude for working with their hands.

Interpersonal Thinkers Like to think about other people and try to understand them, so they recognize differences between individuals and appreciate that different people have different perspectives, and usually make an effort to cultivate effective relationships with family, friends and colleagues.

Intrapersonal Thinkers Spend a lot of time thinking about and trying to understand themselves, so they reflect on their thoughts and moods, work to improve them and try to understand how their behaviour affects their relationships with others.

Naturalist Thinkers Like to understand the natural world and the living beings that inhabit it, often have an aptitude for communicating with animals, and try to understand patterns of life and natural forces.

Existential Thinkers Like to spend time thinking about philosophical issues such as 'What is the meaning of life?' so they consider moral and ethical implications of problems as well as practical solutions, try to see beyond the 'here and now', and understand deeper meanings.

I think I'm mostly a mix between Spatial/Visual, Interpersonal and Existential thinking styles, with perhaps a touch of Verbal, since I'm a writer, but maybe the people who know me best might not agree. The point is that your style of thinking may be quite different from that of another person, so when you're having a conversation you might 'hear' things differently, or in other words, you'll mentally highlight different things. This often shows up in your language. Someone who thinks visually will often use words like 'see', 'look' and 'examine', whereas someone who thinks kinaesthetically might frequently use 'feel', 'in touch' and 'handle'. That doesn't mean the rest of us can't use those words, of course, but we do tend to emphasize words that sum up the way we relate to life.

Another important aspect of your thinking process is whether you generally view things from a positive or a negative perspective. This is often described as seeing things from a 'glass half full' or 'glass half empty' view-point, but from a metaphysical perspective each thought has an energetic vibration, so it does actually matter whether you think optimistically or pessimistically.

THE ENERGETIC CONNECTION

Scientists have proved that everything in the Universe is energy – planets, people, animals, birds, fish, insects, plants, rocks, crystals and even manufactured goods like refrigerators and TVs (because they are made from things that were once natural materials). All energy is part of a continuum from dense, slow-moving energy with low vibrations at one end, which is things we can see, that is, physical matter, to light, fast-moving energy with high vibrations at the other end, which is spiritual energy, or consciousness, which we can't see, and everything that exists has its place somewhere on this continuum.

Low Vibrations	High Vibrations
Dense Energy ⟵——————⟶	**Spiritual Energy**
(Matter)	(Consciousness)

This includes thoughts, which are fast-moving, high-vibrational energy. We may not be able to see them, but their energies can be detected by sensitive scientific equipment. Each thought has a different vibrational frequency, and there is a theory that these frequencies attract people, situations and experiences towards you that have a similar frequency. For example, if you are thinking pessimistic thoughts, they have a fairly low vibration, so you are likely to attract situations – such as being unsuccessful when applying for a job – which 'prove' that your pessimism was accurate. However, if you are thinking in an optimistic way, that has a slightly higher vibration which will attract more success into your life, thus 'proving', again, that your thoughts and expectations were valid.

You may have heard of this theory recently as something called 'cosmic ordering', and there are now lots of self-help books expounding the theory, such as *The Secret* by Rhonda Byrne and *Life is a Gift* by Gill Edwards. According to the theory, everything you think, feel, say or do produces energetic vibrations that attract towards you whatever you are thinking about or feeling. Basically, *you get what you focus on*. Therefore thoughts and emotions with higher vibrations – positivity, joy, love – attract much more of what you want in life, whereas thoughts and emotions with lower vibrations – fear, doubt, worry – block whatever you are yearning for, and keep you in the same fearful, doubting, worrisome situations.

YOU ARE WHAT YOU THINK

From this perspective, 'you are what you think'. If your thoughts are energy, vibrating at different rates, each attracting to you those things to which you give most of your attention, this means that you are constantly creating your own reality, and what you think about yourself is what you become; how you think life is, is what it turns out to be for you.

Above I referred to the energy continuum, which spreads at one end from dense physical matter to the other end, which is spiritual energy or consciousness. Human consciousness is made up of a person's subconscious self, their conscious self, or ego/personality, and their super-conscious, sometimes referred to as the Higher Self, or spiritual insight and guidance. The 'self' can therefore be defined as a continuum of awareness, and every thought or emotion you have is a tiny fragment of that awareness.

⟵───────────────────────────────⟶

Subconscious   Conscious Self   Super-conscious

1. The **Super-conscious**, or Higher Self, is the part of us that we might call our Soul or spirit; our true self that is fully connected to the God/Goddess consciousness and that has full knowledge of our life purpose and the lessons and experiences we have chosen for this life. It is the very wise part of ourselves that is totally loving and supportive, and always working with us for our greatest and highest good by subtly guiding us and providing us with intuition and

deep insight, whether we choose to acknowledge and act on this wisdom or ignore it. (This is the level through which we channel the pure, loving, healing Reiki energy.)

2. The **Conscious Self**, sometimes referred to as the Ego, is who we think we are, in other words our thinking, speaking, acting self, our personality, beliefs, attitudes, concepts, likes, dislikes and so on – everything that makes us recognizable as ourselves. The Conscious Self is not necessarily aware of the helpful insights provided by either the Higher Self or the Subconscious, but can operate independently until such time as a person is ready to begin to discover more about themselves, developing and growing personally and spiritually so that they become more 'in tune' with the other aspects of their consciousness.

3. The **Subconscious**, which works with the Higher Self to provide intuition and insight to the Conscious Self through dreams, visualizations, instinctive 'feelings' or 'gut reactions', and other aspects of the mind–body connection.

Your consciousness, or thinking, feeling self, is constantly creating thoughts – as mentioned earlier, more than 60,000 thoughts each day – but unfortunately your consciousness is often locked in the past, so it keeps recreating the same old patterns, based on the same old thoughts and beliefs about yourself, your abilities, your body and the world around you. This can result in what is termed 'Faulty Thinking'.

Faulty Thinking

At the beginning of this chapter I said that your thoughts generate your emotions, and of course your emotions demonstrate how you feel about life. 'Faulty thinking' contributes to or creates most upsetting emotions, including anger, guilt, anxiety, resentment and poor self-esteem. Some examples of faulty thinking are:

◆ **Black and white thinking** You see things in a polarized way – good or bad, positive or negative, success or failure – rather than considering that most things probably fall in the middle ground.

◆ **Blaming** You refuse to accept disappointment or human failings if other people let you down, and become bitter or resentful.

◆ **Comparing** You compare yourself unfavourably with other people, either those you know, or famous people you've never met, such as those who exist in the celebrity culture of the Western world today.

◆ **Filtering** You filter out or ignore the positives and home in on the negatives of a situation.

◆ **Jumping to conclusions** You assume the worst or interpret other people's motives, actions or comments negatively.

◆ **Labelling** You live with an uncomplimentary label for yourself, such as thinking you're stupid or lazy, or you label others in an equally uncomplimentary way.

◆ **Mind reading** You think you know what other people are thinking, basing your ideas on what you might think under similar circumstances.

◆ **Over-generalizing** You draw negative conclusions

about yourself, other people or life situations, based on limited evidence.

◆ **Personalizing** You incorrectly assume that other people's reactions are directed at you, or you feel responsible for things that are not your fault.

◆ **Predicting catastrophe** You focus on negative outcomes such as potential failure, rejection or loss and therefore make yourself anxious.

Each person's mind is filled with an internal dialogue most of the time – what we call the 'monkey mind' – as thoughts, judgements and feelings ceaselessly swirl around it, and these beliefs and assumptions create your reality, your perception of the world you live in. Each person's reality is different from every other person's reality. In effect, no two people share exactly the same world, because no two people share exactly the same thoughts and beliefs, since no two people have shared exactly the same life experiences – even identical twins.

PSYCHOLOGICAL PROGRAMMING

Just as with the emotional programming referred to in Chapter 5, your beliefs and ways of thinking are the product of programming that began when you were a small child. The way you think about yourself, and your beliefs about everything in your life, from money, work and status through to love, sex and relationships, and even whether you are mostly 'laid back' about things or tend to be a 'worrier', have all been founded on how your parents, teachers and other significant adults behaved, and

127

what they thought and believed. If as a child you experienced a lot of negative programming from parents or other adults who believed that 'life is a struggle', or 'nothing ever works out right' or 'people can't be trusted' and other such judgemental beliefs, then these beliefs will probably inform your attitudes and concepts now. However, just as with your emotional programming, you can let go of your psychological programming, the ways of thinking that no longer serve you, and make up your own mind. You can give yourself permission to change.

I use the word 'permission' deliberately, because changing your beliefs, concepts and thinking patterns can be quite a challenging process. You may have had these ways of thinking for many years, so they have become an essential part of you, but if they are now limiting you or holding you back, then it is time to let them go.

Whatever our thinking style, when we look at the way we live our life, we usually have only one perspective on it – our own – and that isn't generally very objective. Your perspective on yourself and your life is limited by your personal view of the world, your own experiences, the concepts, attitudes and beliefs you have. It's therefore hardly surprising that we sometimes (or most times!) limit ourselves and stop ourselves doing things we want to do, because often we have formed well-scripted reasons why we shouldn't, couldn't, mustn't, oughtn't, etc. What would it be like if you could look at things from other perspectives? What new ideas or thoughts or beliefs could you explore? This exercise is designed to help you to do just that.

CHANGING PERSPECTIVES

Spend a few minutes deciding what you want to work on – think of something you want to do and think you could do, but something stops you, and you would like to respond differently. It is helpful to write down your responses as you go through the exercise, so that you can think about them later on.

1. Write down what it is you would like to do, and what seem to be the things (or people or situations, etc) that limit you.
2. Ask yourself how the situation would be from the following perspectives, and what you believe these people would say to you, and write down your ideas:
   (a) A friend who is accepting and respectful.
   (b) A mentor or guide.
   (c) A curious, adventurous five-year-old child.
   (d) An alien – from any planet of your choice!
   (e) A person who would think the opposite to you about the situation.
3. Ask yourself how you would respond differently if you were 10 or even 20 years younger than you are now (i.e. not 10 years ago, but in the present, at a younger age).
4. Ask yourself how you would respond differently if you were 10 or 20 years older than you are now (not in 20 years time, but now, at an older age).
5. If the situation was humorous, what would you be laughing at?

6. What is the 'bigger picture' of which this situation is only a part?

7. Consider your viewpoint now that you have looked at the situation from other perspectives.
    (a) How do you perceive the situation differently? Has your own perspective shifted?
    (b) What new and different possibilities are there now as a result of looking at the situation from multiple perceptions?

8. Spend a little time thinking about how the whole exercise has affected you, then perhaps give yourself some Reiki for a while, either a full self-treatment, or simply place your hands on your chest or solar plexus and let the Reiki flow into you.

THE POWER OF WORDS

The words you say to yourself, the words that other people say to you (especially in childhood) or that you hear on TV or in films, and the words you read in newspapers, magazines and books, all have an effect on you and on your life-force energy, or Ki. As an example of how words can affect you, try this exercise in front of a mirror.

WORD POWER

Stand up straight and look at yourself in the mirror. Now begin to say aloud the words 'I am sad', repeating the phrase at least 10, but not more than 20 times, and watch what happens to your body and listen to what happens to your voice. Your shoulders and back may begin to slump, you will probably find it a bit difficult to keep eye contact with yourself in the mirror, your breathing will become slower, you may begin to feel quite emotional and your voice will drop and become quieter.

Now reverse the process, continuing to watch and listen to yourself, and begin to say aloud the words 'I am happy', repeating them 10 to 20 times. You will find that your body straightens up, your eyes become sparkly, a smile appears on your face – you may even laugh – and your voice lightens. And all from a few words!

What this demonstrates is how important it is to monitor what you say about yourself. Like the words of a well-known song, you need to 'accentuate the positive, eliminate the negative, and latch on to the affirmative'. I often overhear people saying really negative things about themselves, calling themselves stupid, or saying that they can't do things or that they'll never be able to achieve something. If you keep telling yourself that, you'll believe it and it will become a self-fulfilling prophecy. Just try really listening to what you say for one day, and you'll be astonished at how many negative statements you make, especially as you'll probably be trying to be particularly positive that day. Once you've identified the problem, however, the situation can be changed. You've probably been brought up to be modest, but it really pays to say nice things about yourself and if at first you feel a bit awkward about saying good things about yourself to other people, then say them aloud when you're alone. They still work that way, and it will be good practice for being positive about yourself to others.

WHAT DO YOU SAY ABOUT YOURSELF?

- Take a pen and paper and write a description of yourself. Be as honest as you can, so it's OK to put what you perceive to be negative traits as well as positive things. You might find it easiest to list some words. They can be descriptive of you, e.g. tall, blonde, plump, but try to include personality traits (e.g. kind, generous, grumpy), thinking processes (e.g. logical, a bit slow), skills (e.g. good cook) and abilities, attitudes, beliefs, etc.
- Put a tick against all the words that are positive and affirming, and a cross against all the words that are disapproving and negative.
- Add up your scores. Do you have more positive than negative traits, or the other way around, or is your list fairly balanced?
- Finally, cross out *all* the negative words – you don't need to be self-critical, you need to be self-affirming!

OPTIMISM VERSUS PESSIMISM

Once you've identified that the way you think doesn't seem to be working in your favour, you can change it. Instead of being a pessimist, someone who always sees the glass as 'half empty', you can turn yourself into an optimist who always sees the glass as 'half full', someone who believes that lots of good things will happen to them and that they can live happily.

I know that some people believe that even *thinking* that something good might happen will jinx it, but that really isn't true. If you look into theories of universal abundance, which are covered in some detail in Chapter 10, you will see that thinking, feeling and acting positively can have really beneficial effects on your life. If you can replace negative thoughts and worries with positive thoughts and hopes, you will not only feel better, but the energies around you will be lighter and you'll be much more likely to attract those good results you've been hoping for. Even if you're a bit sceptical about energy theories and the abundant universe, thinking positively will still have a good effect on your body language, and you'll find that people around you will respond to you better, which in turn will help you to be more confident, and so on.

A REIKI TECHNIQUE FOR CHANGING YOUR THINKING

Here's a Reiki technique to help you to rid yourself of negative thinking, old belief patterns and worries, and change your thinking to a more positive and optimistic frame of mind.

1. Sit comfortably, and spend a few moments breathing deeply to help you to become centred, with your hands in the gassho (prayer) position, and allow your mind to become calm. Then *intend* that the Reiki should flow to remove any negative beliefs, worries, pessimistic thinking or unhelpful habits from your mind, and if you wish, you can say silently to yourself 'let Reiki remove any toxic thoughts or beliefs now'.

2. Place one hand on your sacral chakra, which is 2–5 cm (1–2 inch) below your navel, and the other hand on your forehead, over the brow or third eye chakra, and wait for the Reiki to build up. Sense the energy in your hands and hold this position for about five minutes, or until you feel the energy has balanced in both hands (sometimes it is better to hold the hands slightly away from the body, in the aura, as this makes it easier to feel the change in energies).

3. Remove your hand from your forehead and place it on top of the other hand on your sacral chakra. Silently ask the Reiki to remove from your mind

any negative beliefs, worries, pessimistic thinking or unhelpful habits that are holding you back and preventing you from living life to your fullest potential. Keep both hands in place, and let Reiki flow into your sacral chakra for as long as you feel is necessary, which will probably be between 10 and 30 minutes.

4. Finish by placing your hands at mid-chest height in the gassho position and mentally give thanks for the Reiki, bowing slightly as a mark of respect.

Having looked at our thinking processes, and at how various ways of thinking can interfere with living the Reiki way, in the next chapter we look more specifically at worry, and what worries are based on – fear – and how to overcome both.

chapter eight

DEALING WITH FEAR
AND WORRY

The second of Dr Usui's Principles was 'just for today, do not worry', and as we've seen in the previous chapter, worry is just one of the thought patterns that can be detrimental to us.

WORRY AND FEAR

Worrying means spending a lot of time thinking about negative possibilities, and people who over-worry often:

- Find it difficult to concentrate
- Feel helpless and unable to cope
- Experience disturbed sleep and eating patterns
- Lose confidence
- Develop obsessive behaviours
- Get headaches, stomach upsets or other physical symptoms
- Feel emotionally drained

Worry is linked to fear of the future and the unknown, and is often a response to a 'what if?' scenario; to something that might happen, but that nine times out of ten doesn't. If you think about it, you didn't start life worrying – tiny babies don't worry – so being a worrier is a habit we can get into, a thinking pattern that we've probably copied from our parents and that gets us nowhere. No matter how much worrying we do, it never achieves anything or changes anything; it just makes us feel awful. Basically, whatever problem or situation you are worried about, if there is some action you can take to improve matters, such as asking for help, then take it, but if there is nothing you can do about it, then the best thing to do is to 'let go and let flow'. Easy to say, I know, and maybe difficult to do, but what alternative is there?

Fear is often based on negative beliefs about life or the world, so, for example, if you have a general belief that life is a struggle, or that the world is a dangerous place, it will colour your judgement about what happens to you, and will become a focus for worrying about lack of money, losing your job, being alone or having your home burgled. The trouble is that we like to be in charge of our lives, but very few things are really under our direct control. One of my favourite phrases is: 'If you want to give God a good laugh, tell him/her your plans!'

Life doesn't always turn out the way we expect, but as long as we continue to struggle and strive to bring things under our control, we are just creating an energy cycle that makes things worse. However, there's no point in just squashing your fears and worries down. Instead, try to become aware of what you're really afraid of or worrying about, then send love and Reiki to that fearful part of yourself.

GIVING REIKI FOR COMFORT

Sometimes it's just nice to give ourselves Reiki as something loving, gentle and comforting when we're feeling
fearful or worried. The easiest way to do this is to place
both hands over your heart chakra – roughly over your
breastbone – and to intend that Reiki flows into you for
your highest and greatest good. (If you have done Reiki
Second Degree, you can also draw the Harmony symbol
and the Power symbol on each hand before placing it on
your chest, to enhance the peaceful effects.) Even 5
minutes like this will be helpful, but if you have 15 or 20
minutes to spare that's even better. By the end of that time
you should find that your heart rate and pace of breathing
have become slower, and that you feel more relaxed and
peaceful.

WHAT IS FEAR?

If our worried thoughts are caused by things we're afraid
of, what exactly is fear? The dictionary definition is: an
unpleasant emotion caused by exposure to danger, expectation of pain, etc; a state of alarm; dread or fearful respect
towards; anxiety or apprehension about. Another way of
looking at it is to use each of the letters in the word:

False
Expectations
Appearing
Real

Fear is sometimes divided into two types – *fear of the unknown*, because we don't know what to expect, and *fear of the known* because we *think* we already know what to expect, and we don't want to repeat it. However, all fear is really of the unknown, because we cannot accurately anticipate what the future will bring.

Fear, worry, dread, anxiety and apprehension are all wasted thoughts and emotions, because they don't change anything. OK, some fears keep us safe – for example, knowing that crossing a road without due care and attention could get us killed makes us more wary – but some fears keep us from experiencing life in all its fullness and wonder. Some of the fears many people experience are:

♦ Fear of the future – of bad things that might happen to you
♦ Fear of getting old and being alone
♦ Fear of illness, especially cancer
♦ Fear of being a failure – in relationships or at work
♦ Fear of not having enough money, now or in the future
♦ Fear of losing your job
♦ Fear of death

In her book *Feel the Fear and Do it Anyway*, one of my favourite authors, Susan Jeffers, describes several different levels of fear:

Level 1 Fears are situation orientated, and they can be divided into two categories. First there are those that 'happen', i.e. those over which we have no control, such as ageing, reaching retirement, losing a loved one or dying. Second, there are those requiring action, which might include a fear of flying, driving, public speaking, ending or beginning a relationship, or making mistakes.

Level 2 Fears are ego based, and they include such things as rejection, success, failure, being vulnerable, being conned, helplessness, disapproval or loss of image. These have to do with inner states of mind rather than external situations. They reflect your sense of self and your ability to handle this world, so if you are afraid of being rejected, this fear will affect almost every area of your life – friends, intimate relationships, job interviews, etc. The way in which you begin to protect yourself from this fear is simply to avoid any situation that might invite rejection, and as a result you greatly limit yourself and your life. You have less potential for happiness.

Level 3 Finally, Susan Jeffers says Level 3 fear is the basis of *all* fear: it is an inner belief that 'I can't handle it!'

Level 1 fears therefore include: I can't handle illness, making a mistake, losing my job, getting old, being alone or making a fool of myself, etc. Level 2 fears include: I can't handle the responsibility of success, failure or being rejected, etc.

Susan Jeffers believes that all you have to do to diminish your fear is to develop more trust in your ability to handle whatever comes your way. Try this next exercise when you're not feeling particularly worried or fearful, and the next time those thoughts and feelings arise you will hopefully have a better coping mechanism.

COPING WITH FEARS AND WORRIES

A powerful way of dealing with fears is to visualize what it is you're worried about or afraid of – such as a visit to the dentist, losing your job or even something like the death of a parent or partner, if that is something constantly on your mind – and in your imagination see yourself coping with it.

See yourself at the various stages of the event, dealing with the difficulties or challenges it presents, perhaps getting help from family, friends, colleagues or officials, then see yourself at the conclusion of the event – you've survived!

Your life may have changed because of that event, but most challenges really can be overcome, either by adopting a new approach or by getting help from the right people. If you use Reiki on yourself every day to help to calm yourself (see page 138), and you also imagine the energy of Reiki surrounding you and the thing you are worried about, like a bubble, to bring its healing energies into it for your greatest and highest good, then hopefully the issue won't appear so difficult or frightening.

Whenever you have a fearful thought, try smiling, because psychology can follow physiology – or in other words, change your body and you can change your mind. Try it. It's really hard to worry or be afraid with a smile on your face! If you can just let go and stop being fearful about the situation, you'll feel better – and very few things will turn out to be as bad as you've anticipated.

HOW TO HANDLE FEAR

Methods for dealing with chronic fear or worry fall into two areas:

◆ Changing how you *think* about the problems that worry you.
◆ Changing what you *do* about the problems that worry you.

This is what the suggestions and exercises in this chapter are all about – helping you to change how you think and what you do, so that you can let go of your fears and worries.

First Steps

Facing up to your fears can often show you that there wasn't that much to be afraid of after all – sometimes the fear of something is actually worse than the thing itself. Talking to someone you trust can be helpful, too, and usually you will find that they have had similar feelings – we often think we're the only one who is facing some fear, but that's rarely the case. There are some sensible things you can do to help yourself. Make sure you eat well and get some gentle exercise, which fills the body with endorphins that help to raise your mood. Moreover, going for a walk, cycle ride or swim will get you out of your usual surroundings, which is also a good thing. Get involved in some activities that take your mind off your fears, especially things that help other people, such as doing shopping for an elderly neighbour, or helping at a day-care centre or hospice. Hobbies that involve you physically are good too, such as gardening or painting.

Do try not to worry about things late at night when you're in bed, because fears always seem bigger then. Read a book or watch a film (something romantic or funny, not horror or violence) on TV until you're tired enough to fall asleep – if you wake in the night and the worrying starts again, get up and do something instead. Drinking something soothing like chamomile tea (not tea or coffee, which contain stimulants) can be helpful, and put 2–3 drops (no more than that) of lavender oil on your pillow to help you to get back to sleep, and perhaps listen to some soothing music. You'll find that doing a Reiki self-treatment on yourself – the 12 hand positions referred to in Chapter 1 – will help you to fall asleep again too, often by the time you've reached hand position number five! However, if fears or worries are affecting your health or making you feel depressed, do talk things over with your doctor.

MOVING OUT OF WORRY

Breaking the cycle of worry is important. By recognizing how you behave physically when you worry (for instance, you might bite your nails, grind your teeth or tense your jaw) and emotionally (you might avoid other people or feel worthless), you can begin to make some changes that can help you to control your worrying.

♦ If you notice yourself grinding your teeth, for example, you can deliberately relax your jaw and the rest of your facial muscles – and if possible yawn.

143

Yawning makes you take a deep breath, and it acts to relax you.

◆ If you recognize feelings of worthlessness, do something physical to raise your mood. Put on some music and dance around the room, and sing along with the lyrics – even if you feel silly – or go for a brisk walk or do some yoga stretching.

Worrying is often a habit, a 'way of being', so it can be helpful to work out when you first started worrying and why you may have taken on that 'role' and got into the cycle of worry. Did your family worry a lot? Were your circle of friends at school worriers? Was there an event that made you start worrying, such as a member of your family becoming seriously ill, or dying? If you can find the trigger, you can bring a more realistic view to bear on it, and realize that you don't have to follow that habit any more.

IDENTIFYING NEGATIVE THOUGHTS, BELIEFS OR ATTITUDES

Choose one area of your life that you are worried about – for example, money, a relationship, your job – and ask yourself the following questions to find out some of the negative thoughts, beliefs or attitudes you have about it. Many of the words or phrases you will come up with will probably be those you heard in childhood, but some will have become influential because of experiences you've had as an adult. Either way, it can be quite a revelation to find out the kinds of negative (and some positive) opinions you have incorporated into your beliefs, and that are now potentially holding you back. For instance, a negative belief about money might be 'money doesn't grow on trees', meaning it's difficult to come by, or 'you have to work hard for a living', which is a limiting belief meaning there's no other way for money to come to you other than working for it.

1. It's better not to have this because?
2. I'm afraid of having this because?
3. People who have this are?

You might find that you come up with lots of answers, or just one or two, but it's a good idea to write them down so that you can think about them afterwards.

DISCOVERING AND TALKING TO YOUR FEAR(S)

You could select one of the areas of your life that you've just answered questions on above, now that you've found some of the beliefs that could be blocking you, and use Reiki and visualization to help you discover and calm your fears, and to develop hope and trust. Try this visualization.

- You are going on an inner journey to discover and talk to one or more of your fears or worries, so take a few moments to imagine yourself in a bubble of light and fill it with Reiki, intending that it protects you from any harm at all levels.

- Next, imagine yourself on a path at the edge of some woodland, with the sunlight filtering through the trees, warming you and lighting the path. On either side of the path is a carpet of blue-bells, and they look and smell beautiful, and you begin to walk along the path into the wood.

- As you continue walking, ahead of you there is something blocking your path. At first you can't quite see what it is, but as you draw closer it becomes identifiable. It may be an object like a large boulder or a tree trunk across the path, or a person, mammal or bird, or a being of light, but it is not threatening in any way, and you feel quite safe, because you know you are protected by Reiki, and you know it is appearing in this visualization in order to help you.

- When you get quite close to whatever is blocking your path, pause for a few moments, and mentally ask the blockage what fear or worry it symbolizes. Whether it is a person, a creature or an inanimate object, it will be able to communicate with you at an energetic level, so wait until you begin to get impressions and information. These may be words or images, sounds or symbols, but allow yourself to accept whatever is said without judgement or denial.

♦ When you are no longer getting any answers to your question, ask the blockage for guidance on what you can do to overcome this fear or worry, and listen and watch again for any answers.

♦ When you have finished receiving impressions, thank the blockage for its help, and ask it if it would like some Reiki in return. If it says yes, then imagine and intend that Reiki flows out of your hands to encompass the blockage in its healing, harmonizing energy, and you will notice that the blockage begins to fade and become fainter, until it finally disappears and your path is clear again.

♦ If the blockage did not wish to receive any Reiki, then ask it to please move aside and let you pass, and it will usually do so. If it refuses to move aside, you have further healing to do on this issue, but you will have received information to help you with this, so thank it again and turn back along the path to where you first began, at the edge of the bluebell wood.

♦ Let your awareness begin to return, feeling the chair or bed beneath you and the sounds in the room, and write down what you have just experienced, together with any insights that occur to you as you are writing, and any information, advice or symbols you were given by the blockage you encountered.

♦ Finish by giving yourself some Reiki, either over the heart chakra or the solar plexus chakra, for five or ten minutes.

MORE NLP TECHNIQUES

There are several NLP techniques you can use to work on fears and worries, and I've adapted a couple of them here, presenting you with a number of questions to answer. You will probably find it helpful to write down the questions and answers, so that you can think about them afterwards. Try not to 'filter' your answers – just write the first thing that comes into your mind, as this will be the most revealing and truthful.

Step 1
Think of something that you are worried about, which is therefore a problem for you in your life right now.

Step 2
Answer each of the following questions:

1. What's wrong?
2. Why do you have this problem?
3. How long have you had this problem?
4. How does this problem limit you?
5. What does this problem stop you from doing?
6. Whose fault is it that you have this problem?

Step 3
Breathe deeply for a few moments to centre and calm yourself, before moving on to the next step.

Step 4

Consider the same worry or problem, and answer each of the following questions in the same truthful and uncensored way:

1. What do you want?
2. Where, when and with whom do you want it?
3. How will you know, specifically, that you have got there?
4. What positive things, in any way, do you get out of your current behaviour or situation?
5. How will you maintain these things in your new outcome?
6. How will your desired outcome affect other aspects of your life?
7. When you get what you want, what else will improve in your life?
8. Under what conditions would you not want to achieve your new goal?
9. What stops you from having your desired outcome already?
10. What resources do you have to help you to achieve your desired outcome?
11. What are you going to *do* to achieve your outcome?

Step 5

Breathe deeply for a few moments to centre and calm yourself, then look back at all of your answers. Working through them in this way should help you to feel more resourceful, less worried and better able to cope with the situation now that you understand more about your own reactions to it, and have identified some things you can do to change it.

USING VISUALIZATION

One way of coping with fear and worry is to feel safe, and this visualization allows you to create a safe environment in your inner world, a place of shelter or retreat. The Cave of Sanctuary described in the exercise below is within you: a place that *is* you; that only you know; that only you have access to. This is a place where you can go to think, to be, a place that you might like to retreat to before or after any of the other visualizations, and a place that is always with you, if you choose to access it, no matter what is going on around you.

This cave is infinitely adaptable – different images, objects, pictures on the walls, signs and symbols will come to you at different times to help you to discover more about yourself, and to deal with current aspects of your life. Various details within the visualization, such as the speed of the flow of the river, how clear it is, whether the river is young or mature, fast or slow, deep or shallow, will help you to identify how you feel about your life at that particular moment. The interpretation of such features is for you to decide but, for example, a raging torrent could mean that life is going faster than you want, so it could be time to slow down.

In order to experience a visualization fully, it is important to engage all your senses, so the walk along the river and the scenes that follow allow you to focus your mind on the visualization – hearing sounds, feeling the coolness of the water on your feet. Touching the cave wall helps to give you a sense of solid security – and of course you are always in the beam of the universal light to give you inspiration and love.

THE CAVE OF SANCTUARY
You are safe, always were safe and always will be safe

♦ When you feel happy and relaxed, either sitting or lying down, visualize yourself on a riverbank and look down at your feet. If you are wearing shoes or socks, take them off and feel the grass or earth underneath your feet.

♦ Now look all around you – at the grass, the flowers, the trees and bushes nearby. See the river, watch it flowing by and notice the speed of flow, and the depth and width of the river, its clarity and colour.

♦ Look across to the opposite bank to see the vegetation there, the grassy bank, the trees and bushes, and raise your eyes and look up to the sky. Notice the colour of the sky, and whether there are any clouds floating by overhead.

♦ Listen to the sound of the river flowing past, the rustling of leaves, the birdsong, then sit on the riverbank and put your feet in the water.

♦ Feel the water on your skin and notice its temperature – is it cool and refreshing, or icy cold?

♦ You may like to spend some time here on the bank, taking in everything around you. When you're ready, stand up and start to walk along the side of the river.

◆ Notice everything around you – the scent of flowers, the sound of rustling leaves and birdsong. Soon you come to a small stream that feeds into the river. You can either splash through the stream or jump over it, and continue to walk along the riverbank.

◆ A little further along, you see some bushes. You walk towards them, and as you reach them you spend some time examining their leaves and flowers. Then you notice that behind the bushes there is an entrance to a cave.

◆ You feel quite happy about going into the cave, because you know you're safe, so you begin to walk into it. As you walk, feel the ground under your feet, and notice its texture and whether it is damp or dry.

◆ You walk further along the passage into the cave, noticing that there is still plenty of light, then pause for a moment and put out your hand to feel the rock at the side of the passageway, before continuing to walk along it.

◆ Now you notice that the passageway opens out into a huge cavern, and light streams from above into the centre of this cavern. For a moment you pause and take in the majesty and beauty of the cavern, before moving into the centre.

◆ You stand in the beam of light and look around the whole of the cavern – at the walls, the floor, the roof, and begin to feel familiar with this place.

◆ Here in your sanctuary you will find many things, many resources. You'll find a stream of water, of ideas running through; you'll find pools of water, of knowledge; and rocks for strength; and crystals for healing.

◆ Take some time to explore the cavern and familiarize yourself with the parts that are now open to you. As you do so, realize that you may visit this cavern as often as you wish, and the more often you visit it, the more resources you will find, and the more help will be available to you.

◆ When you have explored enough, return to the centre and the beam of light, and you will find a number of objects there.

◆ Pick up as many objects as you want and examine them; see what shape they are, what colour, what size. If you want to bring them back with you, you can do so, or you may leave them in the cavern where they will always be there for you.

◆ When you have spent enough time examining the objects, stand up in the beam of light. If you would like some time to relax and be still and quiet in this place of sanctuary, find a comfortable chair, day bed or large cushion to sit on for as long as you wish.

◆ When you are ready to leave, turn to the passage that led into the cavern and walk slowly out of the cavern.

◆ As you walk along the passage back to the outside, pause for a moment and put out your hand to feel the rock on the left, then walk out into the sunshine once again.

◆ Pause for a moment by the bushes, then walk back along the riverbank, noticing what's around you, splashing through or jumping over the little stream, until you arrive back at the point where you began the visualization.

- ◆ You may wish to pause here for a moment and feel the sunlight on your face, and hear the rushing of the water, before finally putting on your socks and shoes or sandals.
- ◆ Now you begin to notice other sounds and feelings – the floor or chair or bed beneath you, the sounds in the room, any noises outside and the soft sound of your own regular breathing, as your awareness fully returns.
- ◆ When you are ready you can open your eyes and find yourself back in the room where you began your visualization.

Hopefully the ideas and techniques in Part 4 will help you to 'live without worry'. In Part 5, we look at the third of Dr Usui's Principles, 'just for today, be grateful', and at the power of gratitude, abundance theory and the Law of Attraction, to help you to create an even better life for yourself.

part five

LIVING WITH GRATITUDE

Be thankful for everything you have now,
have had in the past, and will have in the future.
Being actively grateful will bring
even more good things into your life.

Penelope Quest

LIVING WITH GRATITUDE

chapter nine

DEVELOPING AN
ATTITUDE OF GRATITUDE

'Just for today, be grateful', sometimes translated as 'show appreciation', is the third of the Reiki Principles passed on to us by Dr Usui, and for many people this will seem a fairly obvious statement. Of course we know we should be grateful, and most of us are brought up to be polite and say 'thank you' whenever someone gives us a gift or does something nice for us. But in order to 'live the Reiki way', I believe this Principle goes much further than that, and what I hope to show in this chapter is that being grateful can add a wonderful, joyous element that can enrich your life immeasurably, so that it is well worth developing an 'attitude of gratitude'.

BE GRATEFUL

Society today, at least in Western countries, seems to have a culture of wanting bigger, better and more, especially of material things – a bigger house, a better car, more money, the latest electronic gadget, more luxurious holidays, and so on – and one of the consequences of this is that it's easy to forget just how much we already have. It is important to value and appreciate many things in our lives and be grateful for our many blessings – to develop an 'attitude of gratitude', rather than just taking things for granted. Few, if any, people reading this book will have no roof over their head at night, no clothes on their backs and no food in their bellies, so even on your very worst day, you still have plenty to be thankful for.

One of the problems is that we get our 'wants' and our 'needs' mixed up. Few of us have everything we want, and sometimes the things we don't have can become a reason for depression, grumbling and comparison with other people supposedly 'luckier' than ourselves. Advertisements for everything from expensive cars, houses and holidays to cosmetics, perfumes and luxury goods are specifically designed to make us want them, to feel less of a person if we don't have them, so we can become obsessed with our 'need' for them, without realizing that we've been 'hooked' into our feelings of lack. But by their very nature, 'luxury' goods aren't necessities – we don't actually 'need' them at all.

To help us to lead happy, contented, fulfilled lives, it is important to distinguish between our wants and our needs, and to recognize and appreciate what we already have. Often we may not reach this realization until some crisis or emergency comes along, and then it can become very clear indeed. Ask yourself what you would try to save if your home was burning down, or what would be important to you if you found you were facing a life-threatening situation, or had only a short time to live? Such questions can often concentrate the mind wonderfully, making you understand that few material goods really matter, and that it is life itself that is precious, and the people and animals you care about that count.

The famous psychologist Abraham Maslow (1908–70) came up with what he termed our 'hierarchy of needs', which is often depicted as a pyramid, with our most basic needs at the bottom.

5. Need for
Self-actualization

4. Need for Esteem

3. Need for Love and Belonging

2. Need for Safety

1. Physiological Needs Related to Survival

1. He saw our first major needs as physiological, related to our survival, so that refers to such things as food, drink, sleep and the need to procreate to continue the species.
2. The second need is for safety, which includes physical well-being, a safe place to live, enough money to live on and psychological security.
3. Once those basic needs have been met, we can concentrate on our needs for love and belonging, such as affection, intimacy and roots in the family or group.
4. The fourth level of need is for esteem, which is about our belief in our competence and adequacy, our sense of self-respect and getting respect from others.

5. Only when all of these needs have been met can we begin to satisfy our need for self-actualization, or in other words our ability to become what we are capable of becoming, the stage at which we feel confident and safe enough to explore ideas beyond our everyday lives, such as philosophy or spirituality. (The stage you are likely to be at if you've taken a Reiki course, or you feel ready to read this book.)

You will notice that there's no reference in the list to cars, computers, cosmetics, mobile phones or any other material goods! Of course, there's nothing wrong with having a comfortable home and some of the luxuries that make life interesting and fun – it's just that we could do without many of what we consider to be 'essentials' if we had to, and whether they're basics or extras, they all represent things to be grateful for.

THE NATURE OF GRATITUDE

Although gratitude is something that anyone can experience, some people seem to feel grateful more often than others. These people also tend to be happier, more helpful and forgiving, and less depressed than their less grateful counterparts. There are a few quotes I would like to share that make salient points about gratitude. The first is from Buddha: 'Let us rise up and be thankful, for if we didn't learn a lot today, at least we learned a little, and if we didn't learn a little, at least we didn't get sick, and if we got sick, at least we didn't die; so, let us all be thankful.' The second is from John F. Kennedy: 'As we express our gratitude, we must never forget that the highest appreciation is not to utter words, but to live by them.'

Well, that is what Dr Usui wanted us to do – to live with appreciation, and Zen Buddhists have a ritual of kneeling for a few minutes, with eyes closed, to think about what and who they are grateful for, and it apparently evokes a feeling of happiness, so that might be something you would like to try.

REASONS TO BE GRATEFUL

Apart from the fact that potentially it makes you feel happy, why should you be grateful? What benefits does it have?

- ◆ It reminds you about what's really important. If you are grateful that your children are alive and well, you don't need to bother about the little things. If you're grateful that you have a roof over your head, you might not need to feel so stressed out about paying bills.
- ◆ It reminds you about the positive things in your life – your family and friends, feeling warm and cosy at home, seeing a beautiful sunset or the kindness shown by a stranger.
- ◆ It turns negatives into positives. If you're having a bad time at work, be grateful that you have a job. If you're short of money, be grateful there's still just enough to put food on your table. If life just seems full of problems at the moment, be grateful that adversity makes you a stronger person.

HOW TO LIVE A LIFE OF GRATITUDE

The thing is, simple acts of gratitude don't cost you much (especially once you get over the initial discomfort some people feel about thanking others). But they can make a huge difference. The simple act of expressing gratitude to someone can make a big difference to that person's life. People like to be appreciated for who they are and what they do, yet it costs you so little to say 'thank you'. And because it makes them happy, it will make you happy too, and that's no bad thing.

Here are a few suggestions for living a life of gratitude:

- Whenever anyone does something nice for you, remember to say thank you, either in person, or on the phone, by email or by letter. When I was a child I always had to write 'thank you' letters to my aunts and uncles when they sent me birthday or Christmas presents, but that idea seems to have gone out of fashion. So reinvent the fashion!

- Have a morning gratitude session. Before you start your day, take a few minutes to give thanks for everyone and everything in your life, either silently or aloud – or in writing in a gratitude journal (see page 164).

- Be thankful to your body for all the amazing things it does – breathing, seeing, hearing, smelling, tasting, feeling, moving – even if you're not completely healthy right now.

- Remember to be thankful for 'negative' things in your life too. Problems can be opportunities to grow, be creative, look at things differently and learn from your experience.

◆ Be thankful that you're alive, and for the chance to start again on another new day.

There's a wonderful prayer of gratitude I found on the Internet recently, and I think it sums things up perfectly.

Be Thankful
(Author Unknown)

Be thankful that you don't already have everything you
   desire.
If you did, what would there be to look forward to?
Be thankful when you don't know something
For it gives you the opportunity to learn.
Be thankful for the difficult times;
During those times you grow.
Be thankful for your limitations
Because they give you opportunities for improvement.
Be thankful for each new challenge
Because it will build your strength and character.
Be thankful for your mistakes
They will teach you valuable lessons.
Be thankful when you're tired and weary
Because it means you've made a difference.
It is easy to be thankful for the good things.
A life of rich fulfilment comes to those who are also
   thankful for the setbacks.
Gratitude can turn a negative into a positive.
Find a way to be thankful for your troubles and they can
   become your blessings.

If you like it, why not keep a copy of this quotation somewhere nearby so that you can refer to it whenever you want a touch of inspiration – on the fridge is my favourite place.

THE JOY OF GRATITUDE

Deep feelings of gratitude can bring about states of bliss and joy similar to those many of us experience when we are using Reiki. Something that Wayne Dyer says in his book *Manifest Your Destiny* is that: 'The nature of gratitude helps dispel the idea that we do not have enough, that we will never have enough, and that we ourselves are not enough. When your heart is filled with gratitude, it is grateful for everything and cannot focus on what is missing.' Wise words!

KEEPING A GRATITUDE JOURNAL

As mentioned earlier, most people reading this book will have many, many things to be grateful for, so one of the activities I suggest to my Reiki students is to keep a 'gratitude journal' in which to write down every evening at least five things you can be grateful for that day. Even if you've had an appalling day, there will still be enough to appreciate – even if one of those entries is being grateful to have got through that day. At the end of a week you'll have 35 things to be grateful for, and at the end of 10 weeks you'll have 350 things to be grateful for, give or take a few repetitions.

This may sound like a very simple exercise, but it can really change the way you view your life. When you develop the capacity to appreciate all you have, you become more content with your life the way it is, and less likely to cultivate the craving for lots of 'new' things. You just view things differently. That's not to say you don't want to improve things – often the appreciation for something makes you want to make it even better. For example, if you begin to really appreciate and feel grateful for the home you live in, instead of wanting to move to somewhere bigger or different in some other way, you will often want to carry out home improvements to make your current home feel cosier and more comfortable – perhaps doing a really good 'clutter clear', or some decorating, or making new curtains or buying fresh flowers for some of the rooms. That way you build in even more things to be grateful for.

It isn't just 'things' we can be grateful for. What about the beauty of a sunset, the perfume of a flower, the joy and laughter of a child at play, the warmth of a loving hug, the delicious taste and aroma of something as simple as a piece of fruit? Taking pleasure in the many simple things that are part of our lives is a fundamental step towards developing that 'attitude of gratitude'. Perhaps we could learn a lesson or two about gratitude and simplicity from the Shakers, the religious communal sect that flourished in America during the mid-19th century. They prayed each morning for the grace that would enable them to express their love and appreciation of God through their daily tasks, however simple and mundane those tasks might be. This helped them to be content with their lives.

Listing Your Blessings

Imagine how empty your life would be without the people and pets you care about, the home you live in, the everyday objects that make your life easier, or the hobbies and activities that fill your life with interest. Maybe you could make a list of the people and things in your life you most care about, and just spend a few moments actually visualizing what your life would be like without them. If you get upset just thinking about it, think how awful it would be if it really happened. That's reason enough to develop an attitude of gratitude, to be fully appreciative of everything and everyone in your life.

HOW TO BE GRATEFUL

Being grateful is like most other things – if it isn't currently central in your life, it might take a bit of practice, so here are some ideas on how to cultivate that attitude of gratitude.

1. Be willing to express your gratitude and appreciation to the people you care about: tell them regularly that you love them; thank them for the things they do for you; enjoy giving them little gifts that will please them and show them how much you care.

2. Practise small acts of kindness to other people too, as an expression of gratitude for the part they play in your life. Say something complimentary to the waitress who brings your coffee; take a home-baked cake around to a neighbour for no particular reason; smile at the bus driver when you pay your fare; say 'thank

you' when the shop assistant hands you your goods.

3. When you notice yourself about to complain, stop for a moment and realize that most people are doing the best they can, it's just that at this moment in time they're not fulfilling your expectations. And sometimes we find fault with others because we're ashamed of the same kind of faults in ourselves, so instead, appreciate that maybe this is just one of the lessons you have to learn, and just 'grin and bear it'.

4. Develop an awareness that everything you 'own' — your home, clothes, car, etc — owes its existence to other people: the builders, tailors, car workers and so on. Appreciate the web of life that brings you the things you need, and be grateful for it.

5. Take notice of what is happening in your life, and be grateful for all the little miracles that can make up any day: the beauty of a rainbow, the smell of freshly baked bread as you walk past the bakery, an overheard joke, the fact that you managed to catch that train when you thought you would miss it.

6. Learn from and be grateful for the hard lessons too — because each time you encounter difficulties and over-come them, you grow. There are ups and downs, happiness and sadness, in everyone's life, but every experience is valuable because it helps to make you who you are.

7. Begin and end every day with an expression of grati-tude and thanksgiving for the precious gift of another day of life on this amazing, wondrous planet. We live in a world where there are so many opportunities, so many possibilities, where we are surrounded by so much beauty, so much love. Sure, we could remember

the negative side of life, but it's so much better, and so much more fun, to be positive. This is about developing an awareness of life and what it means to live it.

THE UNIVERSAL LAW OF ABUNDANCE

According to metaphysical thinking, despite indications to the contrary the Universe is actually totally abundant, and we can all share in that abundance, if we choose to believe in it and bring it into our lives with our thoughts and actions. It isn't the only reason why we should become grateful and appreciative, but the Law of Abundance says that the more gratitude you demonstrate, the more abundance the Universe will shower on you, because you are thinking positively, and positive thought energy attracts positive things.

- Try writing 'thank you' on the back of every cheque you write; pay your bills willingly, with a sense of gratitude, rather than grumbling about the cost.
- Give generously of your time and money to charities you want to support.
- Say 'thank you' every time you eat, to the Earth, the plants and creatures, and the people who have helped to supply your food (and maybe offer an energy exchange by giving Reiki to your food as part of that act of gratitude).

One of the good things about developing the habit of being grateful is that you will naturally begin to feel happier and less concerned about what you haven't got, so when the Universe does shower you with its abundance it feels even more special.

Using Reiki

You can use Reiki and affirmations to help you to learn to trust in the abundance of the Universe and to develop your own belief in your deservingness of love, beauty, peace and anything else you need or desire.

Sit quietly and centre yourself, breathing deeply and evenly, and intend to draw in Reiki through your crown chakra until it fills the whole of your body, and you can feel it tingling in your hands. Place your hands on or near your base chakra and begin to speak any of the following affirmations out loud (or come up with some of your own). Repeat the same affirmation at least 20 times, *intending* that Reiki's healing energy flow into the affirmation to bring its energetic vibrations into harmony with your own vibrations, for your highest and greatest good, that is, to attract what you desire, providing it is for your highest and greatest good.

- I deserve love and I attract loving respect from everyone I meet.
- My life is filled with love, beauty and peace.
- The Universe is totally abundant, and it showers me with good.
- I love myself, I love my life and all is well in my world.

- ◆ I now attract to myself all that I need and all that I desire, for my highest good.
- ◆ I love and appreciate all that I have, and I recognize that I already have so much to be grateful for.
- ◆ I am grateful for all the people in my life, and for all the lessons they help me to learn.
- ◆ End with a gassho (hands in prayer position in front of your chest), and of course remember to thank Reiki for its help.

So just for today, show appreciation and give thanks for your many blessings. I hope this chapter has given you a few ideas to try, to help you to live with Usui's Principle 'just for today, be grateful'. In the next chapter we look in greater detail at abundance theory – or cosmic ordering – and expand on the idea of the Universal Law of Attraction.

chapter ten

COSMIC ORDERING AND THE UNIVERSAL LAW OF ATTRACTION

You've probably heard about the Cosmic Ordering Service – a number of celebrities reportedly believe it is working for them, and several books have recently been published about it. Well, it's all about abundance thinking and the Law of Attraction. It ties in with 'living the Reiki way' because Dr Usui wanted us to learn to be grateful and appreciate what we have, and as you will see later in this chapter, the more grateful you are, the more abundant your life can become.

I've been working with abundance thinking – or cosmic ordering – for about 12 years, and I'm definitely getting better at it. I've manifested (brought into my life) lots of things, often within just a few days of asking for them, so I'm convinced that the ideas I discuss in this chapter really work. Let me give you a few examples:

◆ When I became a Reiki Master I felt I needed a really good therapy couch, but didn't think I could afford one, so I 'put out to the Universe' for one. A few days later someone called to say they would like to take

Second Degree training with me, but they didn't have much money, so would I take a therapy couch in exchange? Naturally I said 'yes, thank you'!

- When I left work I only had an old computer and needed a more up-to-date one, and a good printer, to help me run my Reiki practice, but with far less money coming in I wasn't sure I could buy them. A few days later my son rang me and said he realized I needed more modern computing facilities, and he had a spare computer and a laser printer, which I could borrow. Again, I said 'yes, thank you'.

- More recently, when I wanted to move to the Cotswolds, I 'put out to the Universe' for a three-bedroom bungalow so that I could have a spare room and an office, plus a nice kitchen and bathroom, a conservatory, a secluded garden and views of hills. The very first place I looked at was exactly what I wanted, so that's where I now live. It's not absolutely perfect – I forgot to specify space for a freezer and dishwasher in the kitchen – but I love it!

I could give you many more examples, but that's probably enough for now – and the point is, everything was achieved easily and effortlessly.

THE LAW OF ATTRACTION

I introduced this idea in Chapter 5, when I mentioned the teachings of Abraham in the book *Ask and It Is Given*, and again in Chapter 9. We know there are universal laws that govern the way the Universe works, like the Law of

Gravity, for instance. Well, you may not have heard of it before, but the Law of Attraction is one of the universal laws that is working in your life right now – and always has been. It's as impartial and as constant as the Law of Gravity. You wouldn't expect only a few of us to be affected by the Law of Gravity – it would be a bit strange if the rest of humanity floated off into space! Equally, the Law of Attraction works for everyone, at all times, attracting into their lives whatever they focus on most, whether that is positive or negative.

As mentioned in Chapter 7, everything in the Universe vibrates and is moving, and according to the Law of Attraction, when something vibrates at a particular frequency, it attracts and resonates with other things vibrating at the same frequency. Thoughts as well as objects have their own vibrations, so you attract particular events towards you, according to the frequency of the vibration of your thoughts. The energy of everything you think, say or do draws the corresponding vibration to you. Thoughts become things.

You are basically a magnet. You attract with both conscious and unconscious thoughts, so you draw to you the people in your life, your home, job, car, wealth or debt, etc. So people who think negatively attract negative things. A relative of mine is convinced that everything electrical, electronic or mechanical he buys will go wrong – and guess what, it does. Another friend is always saying that she has disastrous holidays – and she comes back with tales of dreadful accommodation, meals that gave her stomach upsets, and often a bandaged or plastered limb as evidence of a fall.

Working with the Law of Attraction

Because the Law of Attraction grants our every command, the process of working with it is fairly simple:

ASK → BELIEVE → RECEIVE

ASK Decide, in as much detail as possible, what you want to have, be or do, and get a clear picture of it in your mind.

BELIEVE It is important to believe that you will receive, and that what you want is yours already, on an energetic level. You must imagine, pretend and act as if, make-believe, speak and think as though you have already received what you've asked for. When you give out the frequency of having received it, the Law of Attraction moves people, events and circumstances for you to receive.

RECEIVE It is equally important that you feel good about yourself, believe that you deserve to have what you have asked for and think about all the advantages it will bring you. Feel the way you will feel once your desire has manifested, and be ready for it. Be grateful, *feel* grateful, for it in advance.

How to Send Your Cosmic Order

So if the cosmic ordering process is Ask, Believe, Receive – how do you go about asking?

◆ State your intention verbally: say aloud what you wish for, then 'I intend that this cosmic order is now realized in the most positive way possible.'

◆ Visualize yourself in the future, as fully as possible,

with whatever you want already realized.

- Write down your cosmic order on a piece of paper and place it on an 'abundance board' – a small cork board will do, decorated with a few attractive pictures or postcards, or coloured ribbons.
- Alternatively write down your cosmic order and burn the paper, and see the Universe taking care of the ash and smoke, turning it into what you want in your life.
- You can ask your guardian angel to deliver it to you, if you feel happy to believe in angels.
- Make an altar somewhere in your home – just a small space with a candle, some fresh flowers, perhaps a few crystals and an incense stick will be fine – and place your written order on it.
- Write your cosmic order on something like a Post-it note, and hold it between your hands for at least five minutes a day, allowing Reiki to flow into it, for your highest and greatest good.
- Clean a quartz crystal by holding it under running water, hold the crystal in your hands and fill it with Reiki for a few minutes, then place the crystal on your Post-it note with your cosmic order written on it. Recleanse the crystal and refill it with Reiki about once a week, until what you want has manifested – or until you've changed your mind and decided you don't actually need it any more.

There are several things I need to point out. First, once you have placed your cosmic order, apart from sometimes visualizing yourself as if you'd already achieved it, leave it to the Universe to sort out – don't let any doubtful thoughts come into your mind, because as soon as you do, you halt the process. Also, 'God helps those who help themselves', or in other words, to get what you want takes some effort from you, too. Yes, the Law of Attraction will work for you, but just sitting at home waiting for a lottery win won't work if you haven't bought a ticket! Energy flows where your attention goes, so don't just *think* about what you want, *do* something too. If you want to go on a world cruise, get the brochures and plan your trip. (This doesn't mean you should book an expensive trip using your credit card, unless you can be reasonably sure you can pay the money back – with the Law of Attraction, things should come easily and effortlessly, not put you into debt.) If you want to live in the countryside, take a few trips to the area you like best, browse through the property pages of the local newspapers, and imagine yourself living there, shopping locally, eating in local restaurants, and so on. That's living 'as if' you already have what you want, and that will activate the Law of Attraction to bring it to you.

Taking Advantage of Synchronicity

What you will often find is that the Universe gives you signals that you're on the right track – something we call synchronicity. Maybe you see a competition where the prize is a world cruise. Enter it! Or you see a free course offered that would help you to get the qualifications you need for the job you've always wanted. Go for it! Or the company you work for offers you a transfer to the very place you want to live. Take it! Because sometimes the Law of Attraction brings you things in stages, rather than all at once, be prepared to be flexible. Don't turn down something because it isn't absolutely 'perfect', because it just might be the stepping stone you need.

As I've said, cosmic ordering is really quite a simple process, but perhaps you need to practise it? Here is an NLP exercise to help.

STEP INTO THE FUTURE

1. Spend a few moments deciding on something you would like in your life. It could be something material, like a new car, a holiday or a big fridge-freezer. Or it could be a new loving relationship, a successful Reiki practice or anything else.

2. Now stand up, close your eyes and think about what your life is like *without* what you'd like to manifest. Get a real picture of how that is in your head.

3. Step to your left and think about what your life will be like when you have manifested what you want. Really *feel* it. Get as vivid a picture in your head as possible. Imagine everything you can about having this. Use all your senses to connect with it. See it, hear it, touch it, even smell and taste it, if that's possible. Really be with it now. Allow yourself to be filled with excitement and happiness because you have created what you wanted to have, do or be.

4. Open your eyes and step to your right, back where you started, in the present. Close your eyes again for a moment, and remember what your future life was like. Does it seem more possible now? Does it

---

make you feel happier, or more contented, knowing that it is there, somewhere in the future?

5. Open your eyes again, and spend a few moments thinking about what you have just experienced, and *know* for certain that now that you have placed your 'cosmic order', it *will* come, in time, provided you still want it.

Timing

That brings up another point. How long does it take before your cosmic order is delivered? Well, it takes no time at all for the Universe to manifest what you want, because although we live a temporal existence as physical beings, in terms of the Universe all time is now, so the moment you place your cosmic order, it is ready to be delivered. Any time delay you experience is due to your delay in getting to the place of believing, knowing and feeling that you already have it. You need to get yourself on the frequency of what you want, and then it will appear – so this can take hours, days, weeks, months or even years.

Alternatively, it might simply not be the right time for you. About eight years ago I had a dream to develop my own Reiki training centre, and at the time I was living in the Lake District. One day I was driving along a country lane and saw a large barn conversion with an agent's sign outside. I walked around the building and looked inside the only window that I could access easily, and thought it looked ideal to develop into my centre – it was in a beautiful, peaceful location with fabulous views across the Lune

Valley. I drove straight to the agents who were dealing with it, but discovered that it had already gone. While I was very disappointed, I believe that 'everything is as it should be', so I decided that perhaps the timing wasn't right – I had other commitments and responsibilities at that time – so I just shrugged my shoulders and got on with life. However, every time I drove past it, I kept thinking what a wonderful place it would be to use for teaching Reiki (so I was putting that thought out to the Universe). Three years later I found that it was available again, and yes, that time I was able to get it. I moved in and ran it as the Quest Centre for four years, until I decided that, although I loved it, it was time to move on. I now live in the Cotswolds, and use other people's premises for teaching purposes, because that is what feels right for me now.

Another aspect of that success was that the building was worth about three-quarters of a million pounds, which was far more money than I have ever had (so far!), but I didn't put any limits on how I could live and work in such a beautiful place. I didn't wonder how I could get the money to buy a suitable building – I let the Universe sort that out, which it did. The barn conversion wasn't available for purchase as it was part of a large estate, so it was offered on a business and residential rental lease. Initially that lease was more money than I felt I could reasonably afford, so I made a cheeky offer – and it was accepted!

Basically, it's as easy for the Universe to manifest £10 as it is to manifest £1,000,000, so while I haven't won the lottery yet, I always have enough to live a lovely life – because I believe I deserve it, and that whatever I want or need will come to me.

DON'T THINK NEGATIVELY

One thing to be aware of is that the Law of Attraction doesn't recognize the words 'don't' or 'not' or 'no', so if you constantly think about things you don't want, it will continue to deliver what you're concentrating on, i.e. more of what you don't want. If you're thinking 'I don't want to catch a cold', the Universe reads that as 'I want to catch a cold', or if you're thinking 'I need more money' the Universe will oblige by making sure you continue to need more money. This applies to every area of your life, so if you think there aren't any nice men or women out there for you to have a relationship with, you'll continue to meet people you don't really like, or if you believe you have no prospects in your job, you won't get that promotion. If you have thoughts that are in conflict with each other you will attract a jumble of experiences – the kind of chaos that is what most of us call 'reality'.

You are basically a human transmission tower, transmitting a frequency with your thoughts. If you want to change anything in your life, change the frequency by changing your thoughts. Your past thoughts have created the life you are living today, and your current thoughts are creating your future life. What you think about or focus on the most will appear as your life – so if you constantly think about the past, you will recreate those situations. As previously mentioned, we all have tens of thousands of thoughts each day, so that's a lot of creative potential.

The cosmic ordering process enables you to work with the Law of Attraction and become a deliberate thinker and creator of what you want to attract into your life. You get what you concentrate on, and you can have, do or be anything you want. There's a well-known saying by Henry Ford: 'Whether you think you can, or think you can't, either way you are right.' Another important quote is something attributed to Buddha: 'All that we are is a result of what we have thought.'

The Law of Attraction is really the Law of Creation. Quantum physics theory tells us that the entire Universe emerged from thought. You create your life through your thoughts and the Law of Attraction, and this doesn't just work if you know about it. It has always been working in your life, and every other person's life, throughout history. But when you become *aware* of this great law, then you become *aware* of how incredibly powerful you are, to be able to *think* your life into existence. It works on a global dimension too. The world we collectively create reflects the mass consciousness, the overriding beliefs, concepts, attitudes, fears and desires of the majority of people. The world we individually create — what we think, say, do, experience, who we meet and relate to, where we live, and so on — reflects our *personal* beliefs, concepts, attitudes, fears and desires.

I know these can be pretty mind-blowing concepts, especially if you've never come across them before, and some people find them very frightening, because it turns the responsibility for our lives well and truly over to us. No one else is responsible. No one else is to blame. Equally, no one else deserves the credit. However, once you get used to the idea, this viewpoint is incredibly empowering, because it puts you in the driving seat of your life and gives you the power to change, to become who you really want to be and to live the life you really want to live. This belief allows people to fulfil their potential, make a unique and positive contribution to the world, enjoy life and also have dreams of how life will be even better.

THE IMPACT OF EMOTION

One of the important aspects of this idea is that in order to speed up the possibility of creation, you need to add feelings to thoughts, and as explained in Chapter 5, the vibration of lower emotions, such as anger and resentment, actively blocks your potential to create, while the vibration of higher emotions, such as love, enhances your ability to create. So it is important to begin to *feel* healthy, *feel* prosperous, *feel* loved, *feel* successful, or anything else you want to manifest. When you feel good, you are powerfully attracting more good things to you – similarly, when you feel bad, you're attracting the frequency of more bad things. Love is the highest frequency – the more love you feel and give out, the greater the power of creation you are harnessing, so feeling *happy* and feeling *love* are the best ways to put out the good vibrations that will attract more good things to you.

THE IMPACT OF BELIEFS

Your beliefs also have a tremendous impact on your creative ability. If you believe you don't deserve something, then you won't allow yourself to get it. If we take one example, money, by using the exercise I suggested on page 145 you can see what your limiting beliefs about money might be. To attract money you must focus on wealth, not on your need for money – otherwise you will continue to need it. Focusing on an exact amount can be helpful, too. As I am self-employed, last year someone asked me how much income I thought I would need to live comfortably for the rest of the year, and I specified an amount. Just a few days later I received an offer of an unexpected contract for exactly that amount of money!

Therefore according to the Law of Attraction, if a person doesn't have enough money, that is because they are blocking money from coming to them with their thoughts. Every negative thought, feeling or emotion is blocking your good from coming to you, and that includes money. When you *need* money, it is a powerful feeling, so of course through the Law of Attraction you will continue to attract *needing* money. When you focus on lack and scarcity and what you *don't* have, you moan about it to your family and friends, and are always saying 'I can't afford that', so you'll never be able to afford it, because you begin to attract more of what you don't have. If you want abundance, if you want prosperity, focus on abundance and prosperity. It's as simple as that.

CREATING MONEY VISUALIZATION

◆ Close your eyes and imagine a door in front of you. Take a few moments to examine the door. Does it look old or new? Is it made of wood or some other material? What sort of handle does it have?

◆ When you have really connected with where you are, in your imagination, move forward and open the door. Behind the door is a beautiful room lit by candles, and the candlelight is reflecting on the piles of gold and jewels on the floor. As you look around the room you see that there are also piles of banknotes – so many that you can't even begin to count them.

◆ This is your room of abundance, and everything in this room belongs to you – all the gold, all the jewels, all the banknotes. As you look around you, begin to *feel* what it is like to be rich. The gold and jewels are beautiful, and you could get them made into gorgeous jewellery if you wished, or sell them to make more money – although the banknotes are an amount of money that should ensure you would never want for anything again, money that would give you the freedom to go wherever you want to go, do whatever you want to do and have whatever you want to have.

◆ Spend some time just absorbing these feelings, and know that you can return to this mind-picture at any time, and feel these feelings again, whenever you have thoughts of lack and want to return to the thoughts and feelings of wealth and abundance.

THE IMPACT OF GRATITUDE

Gratitude is a powerful process for shifting your energy and bringing more of what you want into your life, so being grateful for what you already have will attract more good things. However, we do need to acknowledge that we're human, and it isn't always easy to feel grateful for what is going on in our lives. When things are going wrong, or we're encountering difficulties, or simply having a bad day, it's easier to grumble about it. Sometimes having a good old moan about things can feel pretty good, and at least it gets it off our chests. However, if you want to attract more good into your life you need to adopt an 'attitude of gratitude', as mentioned in the last chapter. One of the good things I've found about developing the habit of being grateful is that you will naturally begin to feel more joyful and less concerned about what you haven't got.

Something else you can do is to create your day in advance by thinking the way you want it to go. You will then be creating your life intentionally, rather than leaving it to chance with a few stray thoughts. Just spending a few minutes in the morning visualizing the day ahead, perhaps while still lying in bed, can make a world of difference.

A MORNING ABUNDANCE MEDITATION

At the start of each day, decide what you want that day – and in future days too, if you like. Believe you can have it. Believe you deserve it and believe it's possible for you. Then close your eyes for several minutes, and visualize having what you want, feeling the feelings of already having it. Come out of that and focus on what you're grateful for already, and really enjoy it. Then go into your day and release it to the Universe and trust that the Universe will figure out how to manifest it.

When you visualize, you generate powerful thoughts and feelings of having it now. The Law of Attraction then returns that reality to you, just as you saw it in your mind. Many athletes and sportsmen and women use this technique to good effect, visualizing their best performance and seeing themselves as winners. If it can work for them, it can work for you.

THE POWER OF EXPECTATION

Expectation is a powerfully attractive force. Expect the things you want, and don't expect the things you don't want. Carl Jung, the famous psychologist, once said, 'What you resist, persists.' In other words, from the perspective of the Law of Attraction, what you resist, you attract, because you are powerfully focused on it with emotion, so if there are things you don't want in your life, and you keep resisting them by constantly thinking you don't want them, you'll actually be either bringing them into your life, or keeping them there.

THE LAW OF ATTRACTION AND HEALTH

The placebo effect is an example of the Law of Attraction in action. There has been plenty of scientific research which has shown that when patients truly believe that a particular tablet will make them feel better or even cure them, they receive what they believe, even if what they are really taking is a sugar pill.

It is therefore important to focus on perfect health, rather than on the illness you may have. If you don't feel well, don't talk about it – unless you want more of it! And don't take on the identity of an illness by saying things such as 'I'm a diabetic.' If you need to refuse foods that you know could raise your blood glucose levels too much, you could just say 'no thank you'. Don't feel you always need to explain yourself.

Beliefs about ageing are also negative, so release those thoughts and focus on health and feeling and looking youthful. You don't need to listen to society's messages about diseases and ageing, because they aren't good for you.

Laughter is one of the higher emotions, as it attracts joy, releases negativity and can even lead to miraculous cures. There is scientific evidence that cancer patients who think positively and believe that they can get well have a 75 per cent chance of surviving more than five years after diagnosis, whereas patients who don't believe they can get well only have a 25 per cent chance of surviving for more than five years. That's surely a big enough difference to convince you that positive thinking is worthwhile.

Whether you find this approach easy to accept, or think it is absolute nonsense, it is at the root of mind–body healing techniques such as affirmations and visualizations, and many organizations, such as the Bristol Cancer Clinic, use these methods and find them helpful. Try the following and see how they feel for you:

1. Visualize yourself in a protective bubble, fill the bubble with love, light and Reiki, and let that love and light permeate your physical body, imagining every cell within it filling with love and light.

2. Tell your body you love it – all of it – every day, and thank it for the wonderful job it does of being your vehicle for this life. (Even though parts of it may perhaps not be working exactly as you would like them to, there's a lot more of your body that *is* working, and it needs appreciation for the work it does, and will respond lovingly to a loving response from you.)

3. Tell yourself every day – many times – that you love and approve of yourself. Louise Hay, the famous metaphysical teacher from America who pioneered affirmations and the causative levels of physical ill-health, believes we don't love ourselves enough so she recommends saying affirmations (positive statements) out loud many times each day (at least 20 times). Her favourite is 'I love and approve of myself', preferably said aloud while looking at yourself in a mirror. I would add another affirmation: 'I deserve to be healthy, fit and vibrantly well.'

4. Visualizing yourself happy, whole and healthy can be an important part of any recovery process, so if you have any illness or disease at the moment, spend five minutes or so *every hour* that you're awake actually

imagining yourself happy, whole and healthy. Imagine how it will feel to be like that. Imagine the things you will be able to do – ordinary things like shopping for new clothes, as well as things you dream of doing, like having holidays in beautiful places, or having someone special in your life

Note that you can't help the world by focusing on the negative things either – if you absorb and focus on world problems you not only add to them, but also bring more negative things into your own life. I made a decision some years ago not to listen to or watch the news on radio or television, and not to read newspapers, because they were so full of negativity, and I didn't want to be 'polluted' or pulled down by that kind of energy, so you might like to try that, too. I find that if anything is important enough in the news that I need to know about it, someone will tell me about it.

A THREE-STEP PROCESS FOR CREATING ABUNDANCE WITH REIKI

Abundance isn't just about money; it is about being happy, healthy, fulfilled and enjoying good relationships, so it is about living life to the full. These three steps can be used to help you to attract any aspect of abundance, such as a loving relationship or improved health, as well as a more enjoyable job or a higher income. However, Reiki will only work for your highest and greatest good, so if what you are asking for doesn't fulfil that it won't happen – you will get what you need, rather than what you want. By all means suggest a win on the lottery, but if that isn't right for you, it won't happen!

1. Use Reiki to break down your resistance to abundance. Write down a phrase such as 'I let go of my resistance to abundance' and hold the paper in your hands for five or more minutes, and let Reiki flow into it. Think about the statement as you do so, and you may receive insights into some of your resistances, such as 'money doesn't grow on trees' or 'you have to work hard for a living', which would indicate that you think acquiring money is difficult – and you can let go of those thoughts.

2. Use Reiki to promote an 'attitude of gratitude' for all you have and are. Place one hand on your pelvic area (base chakra) and one near your navel (sacral chakra), and allow Reiki to flow into you while repeating a phrase such as 'I am grateful for everything in my life'. This means everything positive and negative – it is important to feel gratitude for all your experiences, because even the negative ones add something good, such as strengthening your character.

3. Use Reiki to attract abundance into your life:
   ◆ Decide what it is you wish to attract into your life, and create a simple, clear affirmation in the present tense as if you were already there. Some examples are: I am healthy, energized and full of vitality; my job is fulfilling and rewarding; my life is joyful and abundant; my relationships are happy and loving.

- ◆ Get into a comfortable position, either sitting or lying down, close your eyes and allow your breathing to become slow and steady.
- ◆ Place one hand on your forehead, over the brow chakra (third eye) and the other hand on the back of your head over the indentation at the base of your skull.
- ◆ Then intend that Reiki should flow into the issue you want to work on, always remembering to add 'for my highest and greatest good'.
- ◆ Repeat your affirmation as you hold this position, and feel the Reiki flowing into you and into your wishes and intention, for about five minutes.
- ◆ Remove your hand from your forehead, but keep your other hand in place at the back of your head. (You can now have both hands behind your head if you wish.) Spend about five minutes in meditation, visualizing yourself as you would be if you were to achieve what you want.
- ◆ Gassho, and give thanks for the Reiki.

I hope what I have said in Chapters 9 and 10 will help you to create a more enjoyable and fulfilling life, and make it easier to 'live with gratitude'. In Part 6 we look at kindness as part of 'living the Reiki way', and how being kind to yourself and others can really turn your life around.

part six

LIVING WITH KINDNESS

No act of kindness, no matter how small,
is ever wasted.

Aesop

chapter eleven

KINDNESS BEGINS WITH YOURSELF

Living with kindness is a vital part of living the Reiki way, and 'just for today, be kind to others', is another of the Reiki Principles passed on to us by Dr Usui. For many people this will be something very familiar, and probably something their parents and teachers will have passed on to them. It may also seem a fairly obvious statement, because we find that if we are kind to others they are usually kind to us.

This seems all the more reasonable when you consider that, at an energetic level, we are all connected, and as your consciousness is raised with Reiki you become more aware that every living thing is a part of you, and that you are a part of it, and that everything is a part of the Divine, God, the Source or whatever you choose to call it. The realization will come that there is no place for prejudice, judgementalism, cruelty or indifference in a world where we are all connected, all a part of the whole, all one. All people and other mammals, birds, reptiles, fish, insects and plants – and even the planet itself – have a vital role to play and should therefore be valued, respected and treated with kindness.

LIFE AS A MIRROR

It isn't always easy to be kind to everyone – at least, not all the time. The way you relate to other people will be influenced by the following three things:

◆ A projection or a mirror of the qualities you suppress or do not accept within yourself.
◆ A reflection of the way people related to you when you were young.
◆ A reflection of the core beliefs that you have about life.

You may have heard theories about how life mirrors our inner selves, so that what annoys us about other people is really reflecting what we are annoyed about within ourselves. Perhaps it's a disturbing thought, but if you look at the people in your life, they are all mirroring some belief you have about yourself.

◆ If you are always being criticized at work, you are probably critical of others yourself.
◆ If you resent being judged too quickly, you probably do that too.
◆ If you get cross with people who find it difficult to make decisions, perhaps you're a bit indecisive yourself at times.
◆ If you're a bit intolerant of fat people, maybe you're concerned about your own weight, or don't like your own body.

Everything in our lives is a reflection of who we are, but it takes courage and honesty to take a good hard look at ourselves, take stock of our beliefs and behaviour patterns, and make up our minds to change them – for the better.

DISADVANTAGEOUS BEHAVIOURS

In other chapters I mentioned that we are all programmed mentally and emotionally by the significant adults in our early lives, and that our core beliefs about life and the ways we relate to others are usually reflections of, or reactions to, our parents' patterns. However, these negative patterns hold us back. Louise L. Hay, in her book *The Power is Within You*, refers to 'The Big Four' – four categories of behaviour that, if you let them run your life, will impede your progress, make you unhappy and sabotage your future. They are:

- Criticism
- Fear
- Guilt
- Resentment

We all have beliefs and behaviours that were induced by our families, and it's easy for us to blame our parents, our childhood or our environment, but that just keeps us stuck. We remain victims, and we perpetuate the same problems over and over again. If there are negative patterns that have passed down through our families, we do have the chance to break those patterns so that we

197

don't pass them down to our children or grandchildren. Today is a new day. Now is the moment in which we are creating our future. We can be positive about people. We can value people. We can be kind to people.

LOVING YOURSELF

If you have grown up in Western society, even if you are not a Christian you will probably have heard of the parable of the Good Samaritan, and although it is a very old story, I think it is a useful example here, and I hope that those of you who are not Christians will bear with me for a few minutes.

A teacher of the Law came up and tried to trap Jesus. 'Teacher,' he asked, 'what must I do to receive eternal life?'

Jesus answered him, 'What do the Scriptures say? How do you interpret them?'

The man answered, 'Love the Lord your God with all your heart, with all your soul, with all your strength, and with all your mind and love your neighbour as you love yourself.'

'You are right,' Jesus replied; 'do this and you will live.'

There is a phrase there that I think is crucial: 'Love your neighbour as you love yourself.' My feeling is that most people, when they hear that, only really hear the first part – love thy neighbour. They completely forget about loving themselves. They rush about helping everyone else, doing things for everyone else, being kind to everyone else. But the very last person they think of helping, or doing things for, or being kind to, is themselves.

Without wishing to be sexist here, I think it's probably true to say that women are particularly likely to behave in this way – the caring for others is sort of in-built, especially in those who are mothers. Indeed, this type of action has become a normal part of what we might describe as a good life, or as some might say, a Christian way of life. Further, I think that many people believe that lacking consideration for themselves, always putting other people first, never finding time to do the things they enjoy and living life as a kind of martyrdom, is the right way to behave. But is it? Is that what Jesus was reported to have said? I don't think so.

What he said was 'Love your neighbour *as you love yourself.*' Surely, then, that means it must be OK to love yourself? Naturally that doesn't mean to the exclusion of everyone else, but at least treat yourself as well as you would treat other people. After all, Jesus didn't say to love your neighbour *better* than you love yourself! Moreover, surely a bit of practice at loving yourself would mean you'd be better equipped to love your neighbour?

The trouble here is that many people have real difficulty with the concept of loving themselves. Even liking themselves can seem pretty hard. Most of us have some problems with self-esteem, and we're not likely to suggest that we're perfect. In fact, we can usually come up with a long list of what we think is wrong with us – but when do we ever come up with a long list of what is right about us: our skills, talents, knowledge, experience, nice eyes, kind heart?

If you were born and brought up in Britain, you almost certainly have a harder time at liking yourself than do many other nationalities. In our culture it is seen as being 'good' to be modest, polite and unemotional (all those stiff upper lips!), and to 'keep yourself to yourself'. No wonder we find it so hard to accept praise, say what we feel, cry when we're sad, hug each other, admit when we're lonely – or, heaven forbid, actually say good things about ourselves.

One of the most inspirational spiritual messages of the 20th century is a quotation from 'A Return to Love' by Marianne Williamson, and I think it is relevant here.

Our deepest fear is not that we are inadequate. Our deepest fear is that we are powerful beyond measure. It is our light, not our darkness, that most frightens us. We ask ourselves: 'Who am I to be brilliant, gorgeous, talented, fabulous?' Actually, who are you *not* to be? You are a child of God. Your playing small doesn't serve the world. There's nothing enlightened about shrinking so that other people won't feel insecure around you.

We were all meant to shine, as children do. We were born to make manifest the glory of God that is within us. It is not just in some of us – it's in *everyone*!

And as we let our own light shine, we unconsciously give other people permission to do the same. As we are liberated from our own fear, our presence automatically liberates others!

This extract encompasses much of what I believe in. We *are* all brilliant, gorgeous, talented and fabulous ... although we have many different ways of expressing these aspects in our lives. We are *all* valuable and special; every life, every person, has a role to play in the whole. We all impact on each other in so many ways, and I think it's important to recognize our own value, to acknowledge how important *we* are, as well as acknowledging and respecting others.

Some years ago I started to act on my beliefs, because I realized I was falling into the trap of always trying to help others and forgetting to look after myself, so I began to treat myself much better. I learned how to say 'no' when people asked me to do things I didn't really want to do; I also learned to say 'yes' more often to things that I thought I might enjoy. I started buying myself fresh flowers for the house every week, and taking myself out for a nice lunch – or at least a coffee and a cake – regularly. I decided to buy myself a little present each week – nothing too extravagant, but just something that took my fancy, like a magazine, a bar of perfumed soap or a scented candle. I discovered that giving yourself presents is fun, and it doesn't have to be for any special reason, but just because *you* are *you*, and you want to celebrate the fact.

One of the things I bought really helps me with my self-esteem – it's a mirror with a cheeky face painted on the wooden frame, just above the words 'Hello Gorgeous'. I've hung it by my front door, so every time I go out or come in, or just open the door to a visitor, I see myself in that mirror and just have to smile – and yes, I do sometimes say 'Hello Gorgeous' out loud to myself as I go past, and it makes me feel good!

I also began to give myself more time. Time to read a book, meditate or chat to a friend on the phone, or simply time to do nothing. I found that as I gave myself these little treats my 'happiness factor' got higher, and as I became happier it was much easier to try to pass that happiness on by helping other people. It felt absolutely fine to give some of my time to others, even if it wasn't always convenient, because I knew that I would also allocate some time just for me. I wasn't feeling under any obligation, or forcing myself to be kind to my neighbour – I was doing it because I wanted to.

In my experience, people who deny their own needs and desires and constantly do what other people want either end up feeling angry and resentful, or, possibly even worse, develop a 'holier than thou' attitude, looking down their noses at others who don't choose to work themselves to a frazzle in the name of helpfulness.

- ◆ Think of one person with whom you've had some conflict, or with whom you feel uncomfortable, and write down three things you really don't like about that individual, or three things (or behaviours) you wish they would change.
- ◆ Now close your eyes and go within, and ask yourself if there is any part of you that is a reflection of the things you don't like about that individual. Be honest with yourself, and don't react with guilt or blame – you always do the best you can with the knowledge and experience you have, but when you gain new knowledge it helps you to change.
- ◆ Spend a few moments sending Reiki to the situation between you and the individual, for the highest and greatest good. You can either simply

intend that Reiki flows to the situation, or write both your names on a piece of paper and hold it in your hands, letting Reiki flow, or if you have Reiki Second Degree, you can connect with the other person by drawing the Distant symbol in the air over the paper, then the Harmony symbol and finally the Power symbol, and let Reiki flow to the situation between you.

◆ When you've finished, clap your hands a couple of times to break the connection.

◆ Spend a few moments giving Reiki to yourself, with your hands placed on your heart chakra or solar plexus chakra, while still sending loving thoughts to the other person (even if this is difficult).

◆ End by visualizing yourself and the other person shaking hands, hugging or whatever feels most appropriate.

Practise kindness towards yourself and others as often as possible. I really like what Wayne W. Dyer says in his book *Manifest Your Destiny*: 'Make it your own special mission to be kind to others each day at least once, and to extend the same privilege to yourself as much as possible.'

So it is good for us, as well as good for other people, to follow Dr Usui's precept and 'just for today, be kind to others' – including yourself. And remember, *what goes around, comes around*, so as you are kind to others, so you will experience more kindness from them.

In the next chapter I take the concept of kindness to

others a step further, and talk about how the way in which we treat others can build up Karma – or in other words, a debt that has to be repaid in some way, either in this life, or, if you're happy to consider the idea, in the next life.

chapter twelve

KINDNESS AND KARMA

We've probably all heard phrases such as 'You reap what you sow', and 'Treat others as you would like to be treated', and each would seem to indicate that it's a good idea to be kind to others, because then they are likely to be kind to us. This is the basis of the concept known as Karma.

WHAT IS KARMA?

The way in which Karma is explained depends upon individual religious traditions, but basically it is believed that the sum of everything that an individual has done, is currently doing and will do, will affect their future fate. Each person is thus responsible for their own life, and the pain and joy it brings to others. In religions that incorporate a belief in reincarnation, Karma extends through each person's present life and all past and future lives as well. It is cumulative.

The basic ethical purpose of Karma is to behave responsibly, and the tenet of Karma is essentially 'if you do good things, good things will happen to you, and if you do bad things, bad things will happen to you'.

Millions of people around the world believe in Karma, and it is a part of many cultures, even those without religious backgrounds. According to Karma, whether you are performing positive or negative actions, the results of either can be seen straight away, producing a pleasant or difficult life, or they may be delayed – even, potentially, until a future life.

The idea of Karma originally came from Hindu and Buddhist teachings, but was popularized in the West mainly through the work of the Theosophical Society and the New Age movement. It became transmuted into a belief in a kind of good luck and bad luck, depending upon whether someone performed good, spiritually valuable acts, or the opposite. There is also the metaphysical idea that Karma is universal, and not dispensed by something or someone judgemental, that it is about positive and negative *energy*, where negative energy can include things not seen as 'being bad', like sadness and fear, and positive energy can be caused by being creative and solving problems, as well as by exuding love and doing virtuous acts.

Karma can therefore be a logical and understandable way of making sense of good and evil, the different qualities of different lives and the different moral status of different people, without having to involve rules laid down by a higher power. Ill fortune can be best avoided by behaving well at all times so that no bad Karma is attracted. Which brings us back to kindness.

RANDOM ACTS OF KINDNESS

A random act of kindness is defined as a selfless act performed by a person or persons wishing to either assist or cheer up a complete stranger. There will generally be no reason for it, other than to make people smile or be happier. Random acts of kindness can be either spontaneous or planned in advance. They can include all sorts of things, from giving gifts to family or friends for no particular reason, to mowing a neighbour's lawn or taking a meal around to an elderly person, to paying for a stranger's bus fare or parking ticket.

Pay It Forward

In the year 2000 the film *Pay It Forward* was released, starring Kevin Spacey, Helen Hunt and Haley Joel Osment, and it had a profound effect on many of the people who watched it because it was based on the idea of random acts of kindness.

It is the story of 12-year-old Trevor McKinney, who was given an assignment by his new social studies teacher to think of something that will change the world, and put it into action. Trevor comes up with the idea of, rather than paying back a favour, paying it forward. He decides that if he can do good deeds for three people, and they in turn can 'pay it forward' to three new people, who in turn pay it forward to another three, and so on and so on, positive changes can happen.

He describes his idea to his mother and teacher, saying that if he does a favour for three people, and they ask how they can pay it back, he suggests that instead, they pay it forward, to three new people. Then he gets out his calculator, and shows them how this would spread out so that 9 people get helped, then 27, then 81, then 243, then 729, then 2,187, and so on.

Trevor's efforts to make his idea work bring a revolution not only to his life and the lives of his mother and teacher, but also to an ever-widening circle of people completely unknown to him, as they spread from city to city. People begin to help others, and to bestow kindnesses in completely unexpected ways. The investigative reporter who eventually finds Trevor and publicizes the idea so that it can spread even more widely is one of the recipients of a random act of kindness, which has sparked his curiosity. He was given the keys to a man's two-year-old car when his own car broke down. The man took the old car in exchange and explained that a great deal of generosity had come into his life lately, so he thought he could pass it on. So an idea from a young boy who believed in the good hearts of people became something that changed the world for the better – just as his school assignment had asked him to do. It was a world where generosity and kindness became commonplace – a happier world.

The film was based on the book of the same name, written by Catherine Ryan Hyde, who wrote it because she became the recipient of almost the same kind of random act of kindness as the reporter in the story – a complete stranger helped her with her broken-down car. Although it started as an idea in a novel, since the book and the film were released a real-life social movement has begun, not just in the USA where the story is set, but elsewhere, too. If you look up 'random acts of kindness' on any Internet search engine, you will find hundreds of websites dedicated to this idea of being kind to others just for the fun of it.

Don't you think that's an inspiring story? Wouldn't it be wonderful if we *all* did that? The great thing is, when you do something kind for someone, you feel good too, so everyone benefits. I had heard the phrase 'random acts of kindness' a few years ago, although I didn't know where it had come from, but I have been putting it into practice ever since. Not on a daily basis, I'll admit, but every now and then. Recently I was in the local pharmacy, where I overheard the assistant telling a lady that they didn't have the medication she needed in stock, but the pharmacy in a village five miles away had it. The lady was rather distressed by this news, as she needed the medication fairly urgently, but unfortunately she didn't have a car, and country bus services aren't particularly frequent. I decided to offer my help – I drove to the next village, collected the prescription and delivered it to her, as she actually lived further down the same road as I do, although I had never met her before. Why did I do it? Well, it was a nice sunny day, I had some time to spare, and I'm lucky enough to have a car and enjoy driving, so why not? And anyway, I do try to 'live the Reiki way', so being kind to others has become a natural thing for me.

His Holiness the Dalai Lama says: 'When we feel love and kindness towards others, it not only makes others feel loved and cared for, but it helps us also to develop inner happiness and peace.'

Giving Gifts

What can you give easily, effortlessly and happily, as random acts of kindness? Here are a few ideas found on an Internet site, which I thought were lovely:

- Gift of service – do something useful for someone, like carrying their shopping, posting their letters or tidying their garden; or donate to a good cause.
- Gift of affection – be generous with hugs, kisses and pats on the back.
- Gift of laughter – share funny stories verbally or by email, cut out cartoons from the paper and give them to someone.
- Gift of writing – send a 'thank you' note, write a letter to an old friend, keep in touch regularly by email.
- Gift of a compliment – a simple 'you look great today', a sincere 'thank you for a wonderful meal'.
- Gift of listening – no interrupting, no daydreaming, no responding, just listening.
- Gift of solitude – spend some time in silence, and respect others' need for silence.

DEVELOPING LOVING KINDNESS

In a Buddhist tradition, Loving Kindness is the first of four meditation practices to develop the four qualities of love: Friendliness (*metta*), Compassion (*karuna*), Appreciative Joy (*mudita*) and Equanimity (*upekkha*). The idea is that the warmth of friendliness reaches out and embraces others, spreading loving kindness, compassion, empathy and appreciation of other people's good fortune and good qualities, so that ultimately you remain kindly disposed and caring towards everybody, with an equal spread of loving feelings and acceptance in all situations and relationships.

That may sound a tall order, but as with any meditation practice, you start wherever you feel comfortable and progress as you gain confidence in the process. There are recommendations for the people you might try to develop acceptance and loving kindness towards, in stages, as part of your spiritual practice:

◆ First, and perhaps not unexpectedly, yourself.
◆ Then you might include someone you respect, such as a spiritual teacher.
◆ Then someone close to you who you care about.
◆ Then a neutral person, someone you know but have no particular feelings about.
◆ And finally someone with whom you are currently having problems.

There are a number of methods of developing feelings of loving kindness, and you can use all of them or just the one that works best for you as your meditation practice:

◆ Visualization – picture yourself smiling, or the other person smiling at you, and showing that they are feeling happy, and hold this picture in your mind for several minutes or longer.
◆ Reflection – think about the positive qualities of yourself or the other person, and reflect on these for several minutes or as long as you wish.
◆ Auditory – repeat a mantra or phrase such as 'loving

kindness' aloud or silently in your mind for as long as is comfortable for you, while thinking about yourself or the other person.

However, the purpose of this meditation practice is to enable you to develop loving kindness to everyone around you, not just to the few people you have chosen in the above exercise. So take the attitude of friendliness, openness and empathy into your daily life, at home, work and into all your relationships.

USING REIKI TO LET KINDNESS FLOW

You can use the flow of Reiki as part of being kind to others, as well as to yourself. Giving yourself a daily Reiki self-treatment is one way of being kind to yourself, and offering Reiki to family and friends is a lovely way of being kind to them – providing you don't make your offer in such a way that they feel obliged to accept! It doesn't always have to be a full treatment.

- If someone you know has a headache, you could ask if they would like you to place your hands on their head to help to alleviate the pain.
- If they're feeling agitated, you could offer to stand behind them and place your hands on their shoulders and let the Reiki flow until they feel calmer.
- If you have done a Reiki Second Degree course, you could offer to send a distant treatment to someone who is ill (you should have their permission before sending it).

- You could send Reiki to a world situation by writing it down on a piece of paper and holding the paper in your hands for a while, letting Reiki flow into it for the greatest and highest good. If you have Reiki Second Degree, you can draw the Distant symbol in the air over the paper to connect to the situation, then the Harmony symbol to bring peace and harmony, then the Power symbol to bring the Reiki in powerfully. (If you are sending the Reiki to some kind of disaster such as a great flood or a volcanic eruption, it will flow to everyone involved, from those directly affected by the disaster, to the aid agencies, medical and emergency staff, government departments who can release funds, and so on.)

Using Reiki in this way is a wonderful method of fulfilling your commitment to 'be kind to others' every day. There is so much pleasure to be found in the power of kindness, but actually it is one of the most difficult things to give away, because it is almost always returned to us. I saw a phrase on a website that I thought summed this up: 'When we bring sunshine into the lives of others, we're warmed by it ourselves; when we spill a little happiness, it splashes on us.'

Developing loving kindness as a way of being makes us feel good inside, because it brings enjoyment and gladness back to us – and if there is such a thing as Karma, then being kind to others is likely to benefit us in that way, too!

I'd like to finish this chapter with another saying, this time from Lao Tse:

Kindness in words creates confidence.
Kindness in thinking creates profundity.
Kindness in giving creates love.

Let kindness flow in your spoken and written words, in your thoughts and in the generosity of your giving. As Dr Usui suggested: just for today, be kind to others.

In Part 7 we look at the last of Dr Usui's Principles, 'just for today, work hard', both in terms of working hard in our daily lives, perhaps for an employer, and working hard on ourselves, for our personal development and spiritual growth.

part seven

LIVING, WORKING AND LEARNING

You are a limitless being in a limitless universe, with the power to create whatever you want.

Revd Simon John Barlow

chapter thirteen

WORKING HONESTLY
AND DILIGENTLY

There are various translations of Dr Usui's Principle, 'Goo hage me' (pronounced go oh hah gay may):

- Work hard.
- Do your work diligently.
- Do your work honestly.
- Be honest in your work.

But what does it really mean? Each interpretation could be seen in different ways. In terms of 'work hard', from one perspective it could sound as though we're being encouraged to become workaholics – although I'm pretty sure that's not what is intended – it certainly wouldn't be 'living the Reiki way'. Is it about 'doing a fair day's work for a fair day's pay'? Possibly, but there's probably more to it than that. Or are we just being reminded that we shouldn't steal anything from our workplace? Well, maybe that is valid, too, but I don't suppose that was uppermost in Usui's mind, either. No, it's much more likely that he was keen for us to work hard on ourselves, or in other words, work on our personal and spiritual development, but that isn't necessarily the way this Principle has been interpreted in the West over the years, so I'll come back to spiritual growth later in this and the next chapter.

WORK HARD/DO YOUR WORK DILIGENTLY

In our fast-paced society, when we talk about work we are usually referring to paid employment, although 'work' can include all those everyday tasks in the home too. But 'work hard' has become even more a part of our way of life today as many organizations downsize or introduce new technology to reduce their workforces. This leads to a culture of working longer and longer hours to cope with a greater workload for those who are left, alongside an increase in stress and feelings of insecurity. In the UK, for instance, we work the longest hours in Europe, and many people work in excess of 60 hours a week, especially those in supervisory or management positions; on top of that many people commute to their jobs for several hours a day. This inevitably leads to an unhealthy imbalance in a person's life, because there is less time to spend with family and friends, or in leisure pursuits, or simply in relaxation and getting enough sleep.

I think one of the mistakes we make is thinking that 'work hard' means 'work faster' or 'work longer'. There's a really good book by Richard Carlson and Joseph Bailey entitled *Slowing Down to the Speed of Life*, which tackles this problem. They maintain that you actually 'need to slow down in order to deal with increased demands, because when people are feeling rushed and frantic, they make more mistakes, deal with others poorly, burn out and lose their ability to think clearly, creatively and intelligently'. Does that sound familiar? Or do you recognize those traits in someone close to you? As someone who used to teach time management and stress management I can certainly agree with what they say, and I know that if I'm rushing around trying to get too many things done at once I become much less efficient and a bit grumpy.

Carlson and Bailey talk about 'working smart' as the ideal in a fast-paced world. That means 'listening, reflecting, and then acting rather than reacting out of habit . . . It means knowing how to live your life in the moment – doing one thing at a time, with presence and at a pace that lead to balance in your personal and work life.'

They use a really good example of what that means, and they call it 'living above the line':

Visionary
Dynamic
Self-motivated

Stressed
Survival Oriented
Bureaucratic/Dysfunctional

If you are living below the line, then your working environment is unsatisfactory, fear-based and out of control; your employers have a poor understanding of their employees' needs, and there will probably be a high turnover of staff – if this resonates with you it might be time for you to go too.

Living above the line, however, your working life will be productive and satisfying, and you will feel part of a team if you work for an organization, rather than just a cog in a wheel — or of course, it could describe how you would feel if you worked for yourself, for instance as a writer, Reiki practitioner or Reiki Master. (I'm definitely an 'above-the-line' worker!)

Part of this issue relates to the following questions:

- Do you do your work willingly and with a good heart?
- Or are you reluctant, only doing your work because you have to, or because it is the only way you can see to earn a living?

The attitude you have to your job, or to your work in the home, makes a great deal of difference. If it is done gladly and cheerfully, with a loving heart, any work can become more enjoyable, even boring, difficult or dirty tasks. But if it is done grudgingly, apathetically or under duress, everything will seem so much harder, and it becomes a vicious circle — you hate the work, so it feels more difficult, so you hate it more ... ad infinitum!

VALUING YOUR WORK

It is therefore important to respect any work that you have chosen for yourself and honour yourself by doing your best to create a feeling of satisfaction in it. *All* work is valuable to the extent that we choose to value it, so it is possible to take satisfaction from even the simplest tasks, and to be willing to do everything to the best of our ability. There is an old Zen Buddhist saying: 'Before enlightenment chop wood, carry water; after enlightenment chop wood, carry water.'

No matter how much of your life you dedicate to spirituality, you will probably still need to work in some manner to feed yourself, clothe yourself, keep yourself warm and live comfortably.

So if working too hard is an issue in your life – or even if it isn't – sometimes feeling unhappy or unsettled or even just bored at work can be an indication that it is time to move on – perhaps you need to ask yourself some more questions:

◆ What is your role or job?
◆ What drives you?
◆ What are your ambitions and dreams?
◆ How do you feel about what you do to earn a living?
◆ What do you believe to be your life purpose?

As you may know, one of the effects of Reiki is to help you to grow spiritually, and this usually incurs change. Even if you have previously been happy in your job, or have felt settled in your career or been comfortable with the ethics (or lack of them) in your place of employment, you might feel differently now, so take a little time to consider the questions above. Maybe you've just gone on from day to day in the job you're doing out of habit, and perhaps it's time to reconsider and reassess, look at new options, re-evaluate how you feel and consider other types of work that you might find more satisfying and more in tune with the real you, now, rather than the you of however many years ago you chose that type of employment.

Empowering Goals with Reiki

One way of helping yourself is to use Reiki to work on your goals and ambitions, and you can use the following technique for this. Decide what it is you wish to work on, then create simple, clear affirmations or goals in the present tense, as if they were already in existence, such as 'I have the perfect job which is fun, fulfilling and financially rewarding', place one hand on your forehead, the other behind your head, and let Reiki flow, allowing yourself to visualize your life as it will be when you have achieved your goal.

Write Down Your Goals

Another way of working with affirmations and goals – such as getting the perfect job for you – is by writing them down, holding the paper in your hands and letting Reiki flow into them for your greatest and highest good, saying the affirmation over and over to yourself while giving them Reiki for a few minutes. If you have Reiki Second Degree you can draw all three symbols in the air over the paper, saying their mantras in the usual order – Distant, Harmony and Power – before beginning to say the affirmation. Do this for at least ten minutes a day until you achieve what you want – or until you change your mind, because we don't always realize what we really want straight away, but by working on it in this way, the issue becomes clearer.

Think About Your Goals

Yet another way of creating what you want is to work in harmony with the Law of Attraction (see Chapter 10) by focusing on what you want, such as a fun, fulfilling and well-paid job, as mentioned above. Visualize it often, but don't keep thinking about what you dislike about your current job, because you get what you focus on, and you'll just stay in your unsatisfactory employment.

DO YOUR WORK HONESTLY/BE HONEST IN YOUR WORK

Another translation of this Principle is 'do your work honestly' or 'be honest in your work'. Being honest and truthful are obviously good traits in everyone, whether in the workplace or at home, but my feeling is that this Principle is about being honest with yourself, as well as with others. It means accepting yourself for who you are. We often confuse what we *do* with who we *are*, taking our sense of identity from the kind of job we have – or do not have. I'm frequently amused when I attend a gathering of new people, because one of the first questions I get asked is, 'And what do you do?', as if my job title is the most important thing about me. As previously noted, what we all need to remember is that we are human *beings*, not human *doings*. We shouldn't be judged as a person simply by what work we do, although of course it is one of the valid aspects of our make-up. As Marianne Williamson said, we are *all* valuable and special. Every life, every person has a role to play in the whole, and we all impact on each other in many different ways. Society seems to have an in-built hierarchy of jobs that are seen as important and high status, such as doctors and lawyers, and those that are seen as less valuable and low status, such as manual labourers and refuse collectors. But realistically that's ridiculous.

OK, doctors can save lives and lawyers can sort out our legal position, but think what a mess we'd be in if no one collected our rubbish, or worked on building and repairing our homes and roads. We are all interdependent in modern society, because humankind has become collectively specialist, rather than self-sufficient, so we should honour and respect everyone for the important part they play in our lives, because without them life as we know it today would be unrecognizable. For most of us it would mean no food in our refrigerator (and no refrigerator!), no transport to work, no schools for our children, no hospitals for our sick, no clothes to buy, etc. Get the picture? We rely heavily on everyone around us to 'do their work honestly'; to do the best they can, for our benefit as well as theirs.

One of the ways of being honest in your work is to follow your life purpose, and sometimes we already have a strong sense of what that is, especially if we are treading a spiritual path and learning to 'live what we love'. However, if you don't currently have a clue about your life purpose, you can use Reiki to help you to discover it.

LIFE PURPOSE MEDITATION

1. Start by sitting or lying down comfortably, and steady your breathing until it is deep and slow, and you feel centred.

2. Begin to fill yourself with Reiki from head to toe, until you can feel the Reiki vibrations in your hands, and sense that it is flowing all around you, within your body and outside your body, in your aura, raising your consciousness.

3. Imagine yourself somewhere beautiful, like on a beach, or in a flower-filled meadow, or a sunlit forest glade, and spend a few moments connecting with that image with all your senses.

4. Then imagine that a little way in front of you is a ladder, a rainbow or a beam of light coming down from way, way up high, and walk towards it and begin to climb up the ladder, or allow yourself to slide up the rainbow or beam of light. (If you have Reiki Second Degree, you can imagine that the ladder or beam of light is the Distant symbol, connecting you with the higher realms.)

5. As you climb higher, you become aware that your body is becoming lighter, until you realize that while you are still recognizable as you, you no longer have a dense physical body, but a body of beautiful, rainbow-coloured light.

6. As you reach this realization, you also reach another higher dimension, and waiting for you are some wise beings of light, and you can feel the

happiness and unconditional love flowing from them as they welcome you.

7. You follow them to a place where you can all sit together, and they invite you to ask whatever you need to ask. On this occasion you have come to ask about your life purpose, and how much progress you have so far made on your life path, and what else you need to do to fulfil your purpose and your potential in this particular life.

8. Give yourself plenty of time to receive the replies, which may be in words or images, symbols or physical objects, or even charts or maps showing where you are now, and where you are going. If you are presented with anything you don't understand it's OK to ask for an explanation – these are high spiritual guides, including your own Higher Self, and their intention is purely to help you as lovingly as they can.

9. When you sense that you have been given all the information that is there for you at this time, thank the beings of light for their help, and let them lead you back to the top of the ladder, rainbow or beam of light, but know that you may return here whenever you wish to ask for guidance.

10. With a final wave goodbye, allow yourself to slowly descend until you reach the bottom of the ladder, rainbow or beam of light, and spend a few minutes in that beautiful place you have created, remembering what you have experienced.

11. Allow your awareness to return to your body, feeling the chair or bed beneath you, and hearing the sounds in the room. If you feel a little woozy, clap or shake your hands for a moment to bring you back into full awareness.

12. Finally write down what you have just experienced, so you can examine it a few times to gain as much insight and inspiration from it as you can. You may find you have been given a full life plan, or just one or two points, or the first time you do this visualization you may just get a feeling of deep peace – but persevere and in time you will get the information you are seeking about your life path and life purpose.

I'd like to finish this chapter with some advice adapted from an old Irish prayer (author unknown):

Take time to work – it is the price of success
Take time to meditate – it is the source of power
Take time to play – it is the secret of perpetual youth
Take time to read – it is the way to knowledge
Take time to be friendly – it is the road to happiness
Take time to laugh – it is the music of the soul
And take time to love and be loved – it is the path to joy and contentment.

In the next chapter we explore ways in which you can work on your spiritual development and personal growth, to fulfil what I believe Dr Usui wanted us to do – just for today work hard – on yourself.

chapter fourteen

SELF-AWARENESS, PERSONAL GROWTH AND SPIRITUAL DEVELOPMENT

As mentioned at the beginning of the last chapter, it is most likely that Dr Usui's original Principle, 'work hard', was intended to mean work hard on yourself, or in other words, work on your personal development and spiritual growth with Reiki and meditation. In this penultimate chapter I suggest a range of other self-help techniques, too, such as an NLP technique, and ways to connect to your Higher Self, to help you to develop spiritually and achieve self-awareness and understanding, mindfulness, a sense of purpose, and feelings of joy, bliss and fulfilment. Of course, there are other ways to help your growth and development:

- Reading inspirational books – there are literally hundreds nowadays in bookshops and libraries, and there is a selection I recommend in Further Reading (see page 255).
- Learning yoga or t'ai chi – your local library or college of further education should have details of classes in your area.

- Learning various types of meditation practice – again, your library or nearby college might have information about classes, or you may find leaflets in a health-food shop.
- Spending time in nature – visiting the coast or countryside, or a nearby park or your own garden, can all be uplifting.
- Studying academic subjects such as psychology or theology, if these interest you – and again, your local college might have suitable day or evening courses, or you could try the Open University, which has a wide variety of courses at various levels, not just for those wanting to take a degree – and not just for people living in the UK, either, as their courses use distance-learning materials. (See website www.open.ac.uk)

The essence here is that this is a personal journey; it should be what you want it to be, and at the pace you set for yourself. However, it is important to remember that *doing* something spiritual isn't necessarily the same as *being* spiritual. Reading many spiritual or self-help books is only useful if you put what you read into practice.

We're all spiritual, all of the time, because that is what we are – *spirit having a human experience, not humans having a spiritual experience!* However, developing your spiritual awareness can help you along your spiritual path in this life, and it doesn't have to be deathly serious – loads of meditation, difficult yoga postures, chanting 'om' at every opportunity, although all of those things can be great, if you want to do them. However, each person's spiritual journey has to be taken at a pace and in the way that suits them, and we are all individuals, so what suits one person may not suit another. In this chapter I introduce you to a variety of 'spiritual experiences' and ideas that can become part of your own spiritual toolbox, to be taken out when you're ready to use them.

DEVELOPING YOUR SPIRITUAL AWARENESS

Unfortunately many people don't have much awareness of their spiritual selves, so they spend a lot of time trying to fill an inexplicable void within themselves by seeking power, money and material success. But the answer doesn't lie outside ourselves; it is internal, not external, and it is the essence within us all, the wise, loving, powerful and creative inner core of our being that some call the Higher or Inner Self. Connecting with it is easier than most people think, yet without this connection it is often difficult to find the strength, understanding and inspiration we need to live our lives.

Some people's spiritual 'wake-up call' happens during major changes or traumas in their lives such as a near-death experience, the birth of a baby or the serious illness of someone close to them. At these times we become very focused, so the more superficial preoccupations of everyday life get pushed into the background, enabling us to reach a different state. The spiritual awareness of others grows slowly over time, usually through developing a spiritual practice such as meditation or prayer – and prac-tising Reiki can also act in this way.

SPIRITUAL FITNESS

Some years ago I read an interesting article by Caroline Reynolds in *Here's Health* magazine, on how to be spiritually fit, which was about our need to develop a lifestyle and attitude to help us to rediscover the real meaning and sacredness of our lives. We all want to have clarity, inner strength and a sense of purpose in our lives, but like physical fitness, it can take effort and ongoing commitment. Getting spiritually fit means living authentically, being true to yourself in everything you do in your work, relationships and leisure time, and making life choices from a place of courage, love and trust, instead of from fear — which is really what 'living the Reiki way' is all about, too.

Being spiritually fit means living more consciously by being more grounded, clear and compassionate. This helps us to make more sense of our lives, because it allows us to connect with others from a place of deeper understanding. When we're spiritually connected we can experience improved relationships, enhanced creativity, a sense of purpose and direction, a deep inner peace and real enjoyment of our lives. Being spiritually 'switched on' gives us greater happiness and fulfilment.

To get spiritually fit we need to use soul-level awareness, which means raising our thinking to a higher level and viewing our lives in the context of the bigger picture. Instead of just reacting to life in the ways we've done in the past, we can start asking ourselves 'What is the purpose, the highest truth, the soul gift for me in this situation?' This will change things in ways that, to begin with, we can barely imagine.

As well as trying some of the other techniques in this book, we can start by appreciating our unique gifts and taking better care of ourselves, partly by living consciously and directing our attention to the areas of life that most fulfil us and bring us the most joy.

Make a list of the ten things that bring you the greatest happiness, and start to incorporate at least one of them into your life every day. This could be spending more time out in the fresh air, doing something creative like painting or writing, listening to music, spending time with friends, baking, reading or star gazing – or any number of other things you might enjoy.

Make a commitment to doing something special for yourself every week, like buying fresh flowers for your home, taking yourself out to lunch (even if it's just a bowl of soup or a sandwich, shared with friends or taken on your own) or buying a scented candle to light each evening.

Practise happiness, because as His Holiness the Dalai Lama says: 'The purpose of life is to be happy!'

CONNECTING WITH YOUR HIGHER SELF

There are various ways of connecting with your Higher Self, and the simplest involves finding somewhere quiet where you can be alone and undisturbed for a while (somewhere in nature is especially good – a garden, park, riverside, etc), then either sitting or lying down, and *intending* to connect with your inner voice. (Energy follows thought, so your intention sets up the connection.) You may have some questions to ask, so feel free to ask whatever you need to know.

When answers pop into your mind it can initially be rather confusing, and you may think they are just your own imagination, but one thing that can help you distinguish between guidance and your own thinking process is the speed of the answers. When it is guidance from your Higher Self, the answer often pops into your mind even before you've finished formulating the question. Gradually you will begin to trust this intuitive sense more, and the more you trust it, the more guidance you will receive.

Automatic Writing

Another way of getting guidance from your Higher Self is through a process called automatic writing. The method I describe is one I use regularly myself, and it is really quite simple. It involves activating the creative and intuitive side of your brain – the right side – by initially writing with your left hand. (Left-handed people may be able to do it this way too, or they may initially have to use their right hand – it depends where their creative blocks are.) Having a special notebook for your automatic writing can be a good idea, as you may want to refer back to some guidance you received last week, last month or even after several years, so do date each entry.

1. First of all, with your pen held in the hand you usually write with, write down one or two questions you would like answered. You can try something like: 'Who am I?', 'Why am I here?' or 'What is my purpose?', and 'How do I achieve that?' They are pretty profound questions, but you may be amazed at the answers you will get – sometimes people get just a few words, a sentence or two, or images or symbols, but at other times they get page after page of information. Or you can address an issue you are struggling with, such as: 'What can I do to help myself to be healthier?'

2. Next, hold your pen in your left hand and write the statement: 'Activate right brain.' This may feel pretty strange at first, but you may be surprised at how easy it can be. However, if what you have written is barely legible, and you found it really difficult, still with the pen in your left hand write down the statement: 'Yes, I can.' That is just giving yourself permission to access your creative, intuitive side, and it really works.

3. Begin to concentrate on your breathing, and as you breathe in, silently say to yourself whatever question you want answered; as you breathe out, continue silently saying the question to yourself. Then, in the pause between breaths (i.e. when your lungs are empty), begin to write (with the pen still held in your left hand) whatever pops into your head. At first you may get nothing or very little, or even some words that don't make any sense. Don't worry about this – it is just your ego putting up

resistance and getting in the way. Persevere and this technique can result in some amazing insights and guidance.

4. When you need to breathe in again, stop writing, and let yourself inhale and exhale, then during the pause between breaths, continue your automatic writing. Carry on like this until you no longer get any further response to your question. You can then go on to your next question, and the process is the same:

5. Breathe in, breathe out and write during the pause between breaths until you are no longer getting any information.

6. If the answers are flowing easily and quite fast, you have obviously established an easy rapport and good connection with your Higher Self, so you can stop writing with your left hand and transfer the pen to your right hand (if that is your usual writing hand) and carry on. You may even be able to just continue writing without waiting for the pause between breaths, but try the full exercise several times first.

7. You can then either go on to another question, or stop and read and contemplate what you have written.

CONNECTING WITH GUIDES AND ANGELS

If you are comfortable with the idea, you can connect with a spirit guide or angel in a visualization, and there are many ways of doing this. The simplest is to sit quietly, close your eyes, and ask and intend at the beginning of a visualization to meet a guide or guardian angel, then allow your mind to imagine yourself meeting them in a forest glade or on top of a spiritual mountain (for example). If you have Reiki Second Degree, you can enhance that connection by using the Reiki Distant Symbol to connect you. Then just ask any questions you like and wait for the answers, which might be in words, images or symbols (for instance, an oak tree might mean strength is needed), or an object as a gift (such as map to show you the best way forward). When the answers stop coming, remember to thank your guide or angel, then allow your awareness to return so that you can hear, sense and see your actual surroundings again.

Another way of connecting with angelic guidance is by using a variety of Angel Cards. My favourites are the Archangel Oracle Cards and Healing with the Angels Oracle Cards, both by Doreen Virtue, but there are many others on the market. Find a pack that appeals to you – sometimes holding packs in your hands for a few moments while you are in a shop can help you to decide which pack feels 'right' before you buy it.

When using the pack, hold it in your hands for a few moments to connect it with your energy. Then shuffle the cards and either lay them out in a fan on the floor or a table and select one, or let the pack fall open in your hands, select a card that is revealed and read whatever it says and think about its guidance.

Why does this work? Because everything is energy, and each card has different illustrations and words on it that give it a different energy from those around it. Your Guardian Angel (or Higher Self) knows what guidance you need, and helps you to select the right card for that moment in time, based on its energetic vibration.

A PIECE OF CAKE

This is a very useful NLP process that can be used in many varied ways, from accessing your natural healing abilities to helping you to learn more easily, but here we use it to help with your spiritual development – to make it easy, or in other words, 'a piece of cake'.

First you need to create three spaces on the floor. These can be in your imagination, or you can place pieces of paper down on the floor to indicate which is which.

1. A time when it was easy for me to feel peaceful, whole and spiritually aware, or when meditation was easy

2. A time when I found it difficult to feel peaceful, whole and spiritually aware or when it was hard to meditate

3. Neutral Space

1. Stand on the Neutral Space and think about a particular situation, such as your spiritual development or personal growth, and how you would like to become more self-aware and peaceful, for instance, or if you find it difficult to meditate successfully or anticipate that it might be difficult.

2. From the Neutral Space, step forward and to your right and 'anchor' how it feels for you to find meditation or spiritual development difficult, i.e. use your inner vision and all your senses to bring that alive. Step back to the Neutral Space.

3. Take one step forward to your left and really remember and anchor a time when you felt peaceful and self-aware, and found meditation easy and fun – when it was 'a piece of cake'. Step back to the Neutral Space.

4. Step forward and left from the Neutral Space into the Easy to Meditate Space, then right into the Difficult to Meditate Space and back to Neutral.

5. Repeat this process for as long as you wish, finishing in the Neutral Space.

6. From there, step to the space that was the Difficult to Meditate Space, and notice how that feels to you now. If it now feels really hard to imagine that meditation or spiritual development could be difficult, and you feel much happier and more relaxed about it, you have succeeded, but if you want to, you can step back to the Neutral Space and repeat Step 4 to enhance your feelings even more.

7. When you feel you have successfully completed this

exercise, step away from the three spaces you've been using and spend some time assimilating the feeling that now you will find meditation or spiritual development easier – and smile!

DEVELOPING A MORE SPIRITUAL LIFESTYLE

Here are a few ideas for living your daily life in a more spiritual way – but more importantly, perhaps, for doing things in whatever way makes your life happier and more joyful.

- Regularly review what you want your life to be like – the summer and winter solstices (around 21 June and 21 December), and spring (March) and autumn (September) equinoxes, are ideal times for this.
- Make time just to 'be' – time for joy and relaxation, taking a bubble bath, walking in the countryside, quality time with loved ones.
- Look after your body – give it good, nourishing food, plenty of water, some enjoyable exercise and enough sleep, and some occasional treats, like an aromatherapy massage.
- Devote some time to spirituality – daily meditation, reading self-help books, or going on an occasional inspirational course, workshop or retreat.
- Try to simplify your life – clear your clutter, spend your time and money wisely rather than wasting them on things that are not your priorities.

- ◆ Release any old emotions, thinking patterns or habits that are clogging up your energy, including any idea that life is a struggle. Commit to a life filled with joy and ease instead.
- ◆ Raise your vibrational frequency with regular Reiki self-treatments and some of the Reiki activities described in this book.
- ◆ Make some time for fun and laughter, because they raise your vibrations too.
- ◆ Trust your inner guidance and 'go with the flow', allowing the Law of Attraction to bring you what you want and need, easily and effortlessly.
- ◆ Find your higher purpose through meditation, visualization, NLP, EFT or any other self-help methods that appeal to you, and then *live it*.

And of course, *live the Reiki way*:
Just for today, do not anger
Do not worry and be filled with gratitude
Devote yourself to your work and be kind to people

I hope Part 7 has brought some insight into your working life, and given you ideas to help with your personal growth and spiritual development. In Part 8 I suggest a couple of daily practices that will also help you to 'live the Reiki way'.

part eight

LIVING WITH THE REIKI PRINCIPLES TODAY

Every journey starts with a single step;
make today your first step into a better future
and begin living more joyfully.

Penelope Quest

chapter fifteen

LIVING THE REIKI WAY AS A DAILY PRACTICE

In the preceding chapters I gave you a range of Reiki techniques and other self-help methods to help you to deal with each aspect of the Reiki Principles, which I hope will lead you to being able to live in the present, without anger or worry, with gratitude and kindness, and with an acceptance of working on yourself as a life-long process. In this final chapter I add to all the techniques I suggested by providing a daily practice to support you in 'living the Reiki way'. I am proposing this as a practice that you can do every day, but of course, just as Dr Usui began his Principles with the phrase 'just for today', you can decide each day whether it feels right to do it.

1. SELF-TREATMENT

Giving yourself a Reiki treatment each day would be a good way to start. If you place your hands for about 3 minutes in each of the 12 hand positions suggested in Chapter 1, your self-treatment will take just over half an hour, and of course you can schedule this for any time of day that is convenient for you. You can make it feel even more special by lighting a candle, and perhaps an incense stick, and playing some soft music, so that the occasion is deeply relaxing.

2. A REIKI MEDITATION AND CLEANSING TECHNIQUE

This is called Hatsurei-ho in Japan, and it can provide a beautiful, peaceful start or end to the day. Its basic functions are three-fold:

1. To cleanse the outer part of your energy body (the aura) with dry bathing or brushing.
2. Then to cleanse the inner part of your energy body by bringing Reiki into yourself with the cleansing breath.
3. When you are cleansed internally and externally, it allows you to bring more Reiki into yourself for your own personal healing, and to send Reiki out for global healing.

This technique may look a bit long, but actually it's fairly simple and can take as little as ten minutes, or you can stretch out the more meditative parts of it (the Cleansing Breath, and Concentration or Meditation) to half an hour or more – it's up to you.

1. Make yourself comfortable, sitting either on the floor or on a chair, then close your eyes, allow yourself to relax and bring your breathing into a slow, steady rhythm as you centre yourself and focus your thoughts.

2. Place your hands in gassho (prayer position) and *intend* to begin the Reiki meditation and cleansing technique.

3. **Dry bathing or brushing off** This combines loud exhalations (make a sound like 'haaaaah') with rapid hand movements as you brush quickly from one shoulder to the opposite hip, or down each arm from shoulder to fingertips.

4. Place your right hand near the top of your left shoulder, hand lying flat, fingers and thumb close together, and draw it swiftly diagonally across your chest down to your right hip while exhaling noisily – 'haaaah'.

5. Do the same thing on the other side, placing your left hand on your right shoulder, and brush down from the right shoulder to the left hip, again exhaling loudly.

6. Return your right hand to your left shoulder and repeat the process again, with your right hand brushing diagonally from your left shoulder to your right hip and exhaling loudly.

7. Place your right hand on your left shoulder again, and this time draw it quickly down the outside of your arm, all the way to the fingertips of your left hand, while exhaling loudly as before.

8. Repeat this process on the other side, with your

left hand on your right shoulder, brushing down quickly and positively to the fingertips of your right hand, and expelling your breath loudly.

9. Complete the process by once more sweeping your right hand down your left arm from shoulder to fingertips, again exhaling loudly.

10. **Connecting to Reiki** Raise both your hands high up in the air above your head, with your palms facing each other about 30–40 cm (12–15 in) apart, and intend that Reiki begins to flow into you. As you sense a change in your hands – warmth or tingling – lower them and place them on your lap with your palms facing upwards.

11. **The Cleansing Breath** Breathe naturally and steadily through your nose, and as you breathe in, visualize Reiki as white light pouring into you through your crown chakra, into your Reiki channel and down the hara line (an energy line that connects all your chakras from the crown down to the perineum), and through your major chakras. Intend that the Reiki expands beyond the hara line to fill the whole of your physical body and aura, and as it flows around your energy system, intend that it breaks through any blockages and picks up any negativity, so that as you breathe out, the Reiki takes with it any negative energy to beyond your aura, where it can be healed and transformed by the Reiki.

12. Continue this process for a few minutes, or as long as you wish, breathing in Reiki to cleanse you, and breathing out Reiki so that it takes away any negativity.

13. Finally, take a really deep breath, then blow out the rest of the negativity and move your hands into the gassho position in front of your chest at the level of your heart chakra.

14. **Concentration or Meditation** Keeping your hands in the gassho position, imagine that you are breathing in Reiki through your hands directly into your heart chakra, from where the Reiki flows up and down the hara line, and then spreads out to fill all of your physical body and aura.

15. This time intend that you are breathing in Reiki for your own healing, on all levels – physical, emotional, psychological and spiritual – wherever it is needed. As you breathe out imagine that you are breathing out Reiki in all directions, radiating out through your hands, around the world and into the Universe, to spread its healing, balancing, harmonizing energy wherever it is needed – for the planet, the people, animals, birds, fish, plants and other living organisms.

16. Continue this process for as long as you wish, and let your mind settle into a peaceful, meditative state.

17. Finally, place your hands back on your lap with palms facing downwards, and intend that the Reiki meditation and cleansing technique is now complete. When you feel ready, open your eyes and shake your hands gently for a few seconds, to bring you back to a greater state of physical awareness.

3. DAILY CONTEMPLATION

This is a way to bring the Reiki Principles into your everyday life with a fairly short visualization that you combine with verbal instructions to yourself.

- ◆ Place your hands in gassho (prayer position) in front of your heart chakra.
- ◆ Start by saying 'Just for today, I won't get angry.' Imagine yourself *now* beside a lovely, calm lake, where there is no wind, the sky above is a beautiful blue and there is sunshine reflecting on the smooth surface. Stay with this image in your mind for a few minutes, or until you feel ready to move on.
- ◆ Then say to yourself 'Just for today, I won't worry.' In your imagination, create a sanctuary for yourself where you feel safe. This might be sitting beside a tall, strong tree with your back against its bark, sheltered by its branches and leaves, feeling the warmth of the sun on your skin; or it might be inside a chapel, temple, mosque or even your own bedroom or some other space that feels right to you, which you can furnish in any way you wish, so in your imagination you can place beautiful pictures on the walls, and a comfortable bed or couch or large cushion to sit or lounge on. Stay with this image in your mind for a few minutes, or until you feel ready to move on.
- ◆ Say to yourself 'Just for today, I will be kind to others.' Think of someone – a friend, a member of your family, a child you know or a favourite pet – for whom you have strong feelings of love and compassion, who brings joy to your life. Imagine

being with them right now, perhaps giving them a hug or kiss, or if it's a pet, stroking its fur lovingly. Stay with this image in your mind for a few minutes, or until you feel ready to move on.

◆ Then say to yourself 'Just for today, I will be grateful.' Think of your family, friends, home, best-loved possessions, wonderful places you've visited that hold special memories, and feel and know the richness these people, possessions and places bring to your life and to your experiences. Feel love and gratitude and appreciation for them, and remember how fortunate you are to have them in your life. Stay with this image in your mind for a few minutes, or until you feel ready to move on.

◆ Finally, say to yourself 'Just for today, I will work hard.' Think of a task or hobby you really love, which is fun, brings you joy and makes you feel passionate – perhaps cooking for your loved ones, tending your garden, painting a beautiful landscape, wood turning, creating a tapestry or meditating, or giving someone a Reiki treatment. Let that love and passion and joy fill your being; let it spread out to other tasks, other parts of your job that you may not always like as much, but that you realize can still be valuable and enjoyable and useful experiences. Stay with this image in your mind for a few minutes, or until you feel ready to move on.

◆ When you are ready to finish, take a few deep breaths and allow yourself to become fully aware of your real surroundings again, then perhaps clap your hands a few times to bring yourself fully back to alertness.

At any point in the day you can bring the images in the exercise back to mind, whenever life is challenging or distressing, or simply not much fun. If you are feeling worried about something, return for a few minutes to your sanctuary; if you feel anger welling up, think of that still, calm lake and allow your breathing to become deeper and slower. If you are faced with a task you don't like, spend a short time remembering the feelings you get when doing something you love, and allow those feelings to help you to change your attitude to whatever you have to do right now. If you're feeling despondent, think of all the people or possessions you are fortunate enough to have in your life and allow those thoughts to lift your spirits. If you are experiencing a difficult time with someone, allow your mind to bring back the joyful, compassionate feelings you have for someone you love, and remember that each person is simply the sum of all their experiences, so their reaction to any given situation is bound to be different from yours.

Remember that 'living the Reiki way' doesn't mean you have to be solemn and serious – life is meant to be enjoyed, so have fun, live life to the full, share happy times with people you love and bless Reiki for the gift it is in your life. If you haven't yet got Reiki in your life, maybe now is a good time to think about taking your first Reiki course, so you can have its healing, harmonizing, loving energy literally at your fingertips, for the rest of your life. To all of you, I wish you joy on your personal Reiki journey.

Blessed be.

USEFUL CONTACT ADDRESSES AND WEBSITES

Penelope Quest, MSc, BA, Cert.Ed

For more information about Reiki training (Reiki 1, Reiki 2, Reiki Master and other Reiki courses) with Reiki Master Penelope Quest, and details of her books, retreats and workshops on personal and spiritual development, please see her website.

Websites: http://www.reiki-quest.co.uk and http://www.penelopequest.co.uk

Email: info@reiki-quest.co.uk

Reiki Teachers and Practitioners in the UK

For details of other Reiki Masters and Practitioners, and useful information about Reiki and other forms of healing, you can try the following organizations and websites. (These were all correct when going to press, but check the websites for up-to-date information.)

The UK Reiki Federation

Website: http://www.reikifed.co.uk

Email: enquiry@reikifed.co.uk

Address: UK Reiki Federation, PO Box 71, Andover, SP11 9WQ Telephone: 01264 791441

The Reiki Association
Website: http://www.reikiassociation.org.uk
Email: co-ordinator@reikiassociation.org.uk
Telephone: 07704 270727

The Reiki Alliance – UK and Ireland
Website: http://www.reikialliance.org.uk
Email: mail@reikialliance.org.uk

The General Regulatory Council for Complementary Therapies
Website: http://www.grcct.org
Email: admin@grcct.org
Telephone: 0870 314 4031

Complementary Therapists Association
Website: www.complementary.assoc.org.uk
Email: info@complementary.assoc.org.uk
Telephone: 0845 202 2941

Federation of Holistic Therapists (FHT)
Website: http://www.fht.org.uk
Email: info@fht.org.uk
Telephone: 0844 875 2022

British Complementary Medicine Association (BCMA)
Website: http://www.bcma.co.uk
Email: chair@bcma.co.uk
Telephone: 0845 345 5977

Reiki Healers and Teachers Society (RHATS)
Email: info@reikihealersandteachers.net
Telephone: 020 8462 1224

Institute for Complementary Medicine (ICM)
Website: http://www.i-c-m.org.uk
Email: info@i-c-m.org.uk
Tel: 020 7231 5855

National Federation of Spiritual Healers
Website: http://www.nfsh.org.uk

Worldwide Contacts for Reiki Teachers and Practitioners
The Reiki Alliance – Worldwide
Website: http://www.reikialliance.com
Email: info@reikialliance.com

International Association of Reiki Professionals (IARP)
Website: http://www.iarp.org
Email: info@iarp.org

Australian Reiki Connection
Website: http://www.australianreikiconnection.com.au

Canadian Reiki Association
Website: http://www.reiki.ca
Email: reiki@reiki.ca

The International Center for Reiki Training
Website: http://www.reiki.org
Email: center@reiki.org

Reiki New Zealand Inc
Website: http://www.reiki.org.nz
Email: info@reiki.org.nz

International NLP Trainers Association (INLPTA)
Website: http://www.inlpta.co.uk
Email: info@inlpta.co.uk

The Global Organization of Neuro-Linguistic Programming
Website: http://www.gonlp.org or
http://www.bbnlp.com

The Association for Meridian Energy Therapies
Website: http://www.theamt.com

World Center for EFT (Gary Craig)
Website: www.emofree.com

Donna Eden and David Feinstein (EFT/Energy Psychology)
Website: http://www.innersource.net

The Energy Medicine Institute
Website: http://www.energymed.org
Email: emailus@energymed.org

FURTHER READING

The following books are my recommendations from the many available on each subject. I have placed them under headings to make it easier to find the topics you want to pursue, but many of them cover several categories.

Abundance Theory, Law of Attraction and Cosmic Ordering

Boyes, Carolyn, *Cosmic Ordering in 7 Easy Steps*, Collins, 2006

Byrne, Rhonda, *The Secret*, Simon & Schuster Ltd, 2006

Cainer, Jonathan, *Cosmic Ordering*, Collins, 2006

Carlson, Richard, *Don't Sweat the Small Stuff About Money*, Hodder & Stoughton, 1998

Dyer, Wayne W., *Manifest Your Destiny*, Thorsons, 1998

Edwards, Gill, *Life is a Gift*, Piatkus, 2007

Frank, Debbie, *Cosmic Ordering Guide to Life, Love & Happiness*, Penguin, 2007

Hicks, Esther and Jerry, *Ask and It Is Given*, Hay House, 2005

Hicks, Esther and Jerry, *The Law of Attraction*, Hay House, 2007

Horan, Paula, *Abundance Through Reiki*, Lotus Light Publications, 1995

Losier, Michael, *Law of Attraction*, Hodder & Stoughton, 2007

Mohr, Barbel, *The Cosmic Ordering Service*, Hampton Road Publishing, 2001

Roman, Sanaya and Packer, Duane, *Creating Money*, H. J. Kramer, 1988

Emotions, Thinking, Anger and Worry

Blanchard, Ken, *Whale Done! The Power of Positive Relationships*, Nicholas Brealey Publishing, 2002

Bloom, William, *The Endorphin Effect*, Piatkus, 2001

Carlson, Richard and Bailey, Joseph, *Slowing Down to the Speed of Life, How to Create a More Peaceful, Simpler Life from the Inside Out*, Hodder Mobius, 1998

Carnegie, Dale, *How to Stop Worrying and Start Living*, Pocket Books, 2004

Dyer, Dr Wayne W., *You'll See It When You Believe It*, Arrow, 1990

Dyer, Dr Wayne W., *Change Your Thoughts, Change Your Life*, Hay House UK Ltd, 2007

Edelman, Dr Sarah, *Change Your Thinking*, Vermilion, 2006

Fisher, Mike, *Beating Anger: The Eight-point Plan for Coping with Rage*, Rider & Co, 2005

Gentry, Dr W. Doyle, *Anger Management For Dummies*, John Wiley & Sons, 2006

Goleman, Daniel, *Emotional Intelligence*, Bloomsbury, 1996

Hamilton, Dr David R., *It's The Thought That Counts*, Hay House UK Ltd, 2006

Hay, Louise L., *The Power is Within You*, Hay House, 2004

Hicks, Esther and Jerry, *The Astonishing Power of Emotions: Let Your Feelings Be Your Guide*, Hay House, 2007

Holden, Robert, *Living Wonderfully*, Thorsons, 1994

Holden, Robert, *Shift Happens*, Hodder & Stoughton, 2000

Jeffers, Susan, *Feel the Fear and Do it Anyway*, Arrow Books, 1991

Jeffers, Susan, *End the Struggle and Dance With Life*, Hodder & Stoughton, 1996

Leahy, Dr Robert L., *The Worry Cure*, Piatkus, 2006

Lindenfield, Gael, *Managing Anger*, Thorsons, 2000

Mumford, Jeni, *Life Coaching for Dummies*, John Wiley & Sons Ltd, 2006

Neill, Michael, *Feel Happy Now!*, Hay House UK Ltd, 2007

Ricard, Matthieu, *Happiness: A Guide to Developing Life's Most Important Skill*, Atlantic Books, 2007

Wood, Eve A., *10 Steps to Take Charge of Your Emotional Life*, Hay House, 2006

EFT and NLP

Craig, Gary and Flint, Garry A., *Emotional Freedom: Techniques for Dealing with Emotional and Physical Distress*, Garry A. Flint, 2001

Dilts, Robert, Hallbom, Tim and Smith, Suzi, *Beliefs – Pathways to Health & Well-being*, Metamorphous Press, 1990

Eden, Donna, *Energy Medicine*, Piatkus, 1999

Feinstein, David, Eden, Donna and Craig, Gary, *The Healing Power of EFT & Energy Psychology*, Piatkus, 2006

Gallo, Dr Fred P. and Vincenzi, Dr Harry, *Energy Tapping: How To Rapidly Eliminate Anxiety, Depression, Cravings and More Using Energy Psychology*, New Harbinger Publications, 2000

Lynch, Paul and Valerie, *Emotional Healing in Minutes*, Thorsons, 2001

Mallows, Michael and Sinclair, Joseph, *Peace of Mind is a Piece of Cake*, Crown House Publishing, 1998

McDermott, Ian and O'Connor, Joseph, *NLP and Health*, Thorsons, 1996

O'Connor, Joseph & Seymour, John, *Introducing NLP*, Thorsons, 2003

Ready, Romilla & Burton, Kate, *Neuro-linguistic Programming for Dummies*, John Wiley & Sons, 2004

Gratitude and Kindness

Ban Breathnach, Sarah, *The Simple Abundance Journal of Gratitude*, Warner Books, 1996

Clinton, Bill, *Giving: How Each of Us Can Change the World*, Hutchinson, 2007

Dalai Lama XIV Bstan-dzin-rgya-mtsho, *Kindness Clarity and*

Insight, Snow Lion Publications, 1983

Demartini, John, *The Gratitude Effect*, Burman Books Inc, 2007

Hay, Louise L., *Gratitude: A Way of Life*, Hay House Inc, 2004

Hyde, Catherine Ryan, *Pay It Forward*, Black Swan, 2007

Salzberg, Sharon, *Lovingkindness: The Revolutionary Art of Happiness*, Shambhala Publications Inc, 2003

Salzberg, Sharon, *The Force of Kindness*, Sounds True Inc, 2005

Wallace, Danny, *Random Acts of Kindness: 365 Ways to Make the World a Nicer Place*, Ebury Press, 2004

Weissman, Darren R., *The Power of Infinite Love and Gratitude*, Hay House, 2007

Reiki

Ellis, Richard, *Reiki and the Seven Chakras*, Vermilion, 2002

Hall, Mari, *Reiki for the Soul*, Thorsons, 2000

Horan, Paula, *Empowerment Through Reiki*, Lotus Light Publications, 1992

Lubeck, Walter, Petter, Frank Arjava and Rand, William Lee, *The Spirit of Reiki*, Lotus Press, 2001

Lubeck, Walter and Petter, Frank Arjava, *Reiki Best Practices*, Lotus Press, 2003

Quest, Penelope, *Reiki for Life*, Piatkus, 2002

Quest, Penelope, *Self-Healing With Reiki*, Piatkus, 2003

Quest, Penelope, *The Basics of Reiki*, Piatkus, 2007

Steine, Bronwen and Frans, *The Reiki Sourcebook*, O Books, 2003

Steine, Bronwen and Frans, *The Japanese Art of Reiki*, O Books, 2005

Spiritual Development

Myss, Dr Caroline, *Anatomy of the Spirit*, Bantam Books, 1997

Myss, Dr Caroline, *Sacred Contracts*, Bantam Books, 2002

Myss, Dr Caroline, *Entering the Castle, An Inner Path to God and Your Soul*, Simon & Schuster UK Ltd, 2007

Potter, Richard N. and Potter, Jan, *Spiritual Development for Beginners*, Llewellyn Publications US, 2006

Roberts, Jane, *The Nature of Personal Reality*, Amber-Allen Publishing, 1974

Roman, Sanaya, *Living With Joy*, H. J. Kramer, 1986

Roman, Sanaya, *Personal Power Through Awareness*, H. J. Kramer, 1986

Roman, Sanaya, *Spiritual Growth*, H. J. Kramer, 1989

Roman, Sanaya, *Soul Love*, H. J. Kramer, 1997

Ruiz, Don Miguel, *The Four Agreements*, Amber-Allen Publishing Inc, 1997

Tolle, Eckhart, *The Power of Now: A Guide to Spiritual Enlightenment*, Hodder Mobius, 2001

Tolle, Eckhart, *A New Earth: Awakening to Your Life's Purpose*, Penguin Books Ltd, 2006

Walsch, Neale Donald, *Conversations With God – Books 1, 2 & 3*, Hodder & Stoughton, 1996, 1997, 1998

Williamson, Marianne, *A Return to Love*, Thorsons, 1996

Zukav, Garry, *The Seat of the Soul*, Fireside, 1989

SUGGESTED MUSIC

Soul Mates, by Philip Chapman, 1988, New World Company

Music for Reiki Healing, by Llewellyn, 2001, New Beginnings

Music for Healing, by Stephen Rhodes, 1994, New World Music

The Fairy Ring, by Mike Rowland, 1988, New World Company

Index